MW01538584

Naturally Beautiful
YOUR FACE

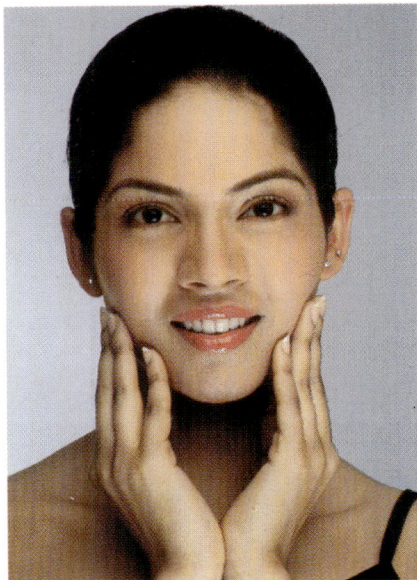

Copyright © Text: Ambika Manchanda 2002
Copyright © Photo: Deepak Budhraja 2002

First Published 2002
Second impression 2004

Rupa & Co
7/16, Ansari Road, Daryaganj
New Delhi 110 002

Sales Centres:
Allahabad Bangalore Chandigarh
Chennai Hyderabad Jaipur Kathmandu
Kolkata Mumbai Pune

ISBN 81-7167-886-6

Cover, Book Design, concept and styling: Peali Dutta Gupta
The Studio, S-94, Greater Kailash Part II
New Delhi 110 048

Printed in India by
International Print-O-Pac Ltd
B-204-206, Okhla Industrial Area Phase-I
New Delhi - 110 020

AMBIKA MANCHANDA

Naturally Beautiful
YOUR FACE

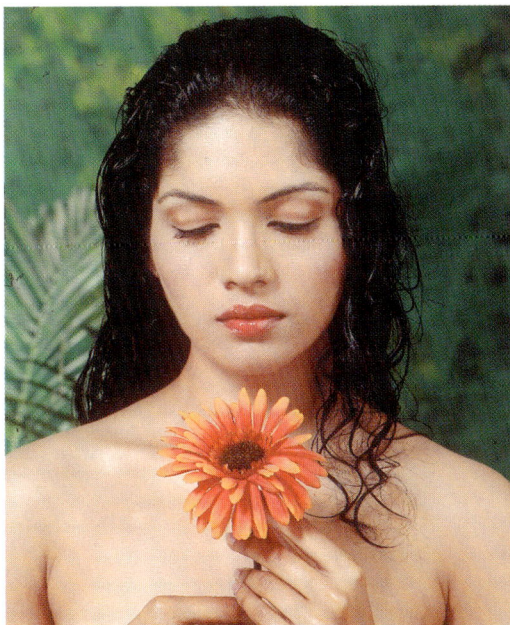

Rupa & Co

To my brother
Patanjali
and my father-in-law
Kailash

Sometimes you love because of circumstances.
And sometimes you love because of situations.
Sometimes you love no matter what.
And that is the best love there is.

Contents

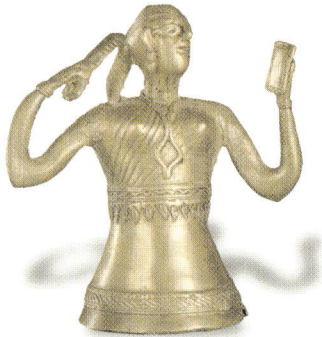

Foreword

Beauty is not the special shape of the eyebrows, the length of the hair, a tiny waist or dainty feet. It is more a way of expressing yourself, enhancing your physical assets and improving upon your drawbacks. Beauty is different things to different people. As the world changes, so do beauty concepts. How did black suddenly become beautiful? And lately, how is it that Indian women have taken all the top honours at the world beauty scene? Suddenly the world has woken up to the fact that beauty is not about looks, or colour, or about how to make up your face. It is much more than that. Its definitely about being comfortable with one's own body. Its about health and vitality. And most of all, its about the knowledge that I am beautiful, because I feel beautiful inside.

Being beautiful is all about lifestyle. Not the way society columns depict wannabes. Its about doing the right things, eating the right foods, and having a fitness and beauty regimen. To do the right things, one has to know what to do. This book takes a major step in that direction. It tells you how you too can be beautiful, with simple and effective directions. The remedies could well take you back on a nostalgia trip. We go back to nature and its bounty. It's a fresh look at grandma's recipes, and the kitchen. A plethora of beauty aids and treatments; easy to make and simple to use. And the results? Wait and see.

Oriental women from China and India as well as those from ancient Egypt were superbly skilled in the art of repairing the ravages of time. They made lavish use of flowers, herbs and resins for making applications and potions that made their skin glow. The ancient art of make-up, face care, and beautifying the body were far more elaborate and advanced than today.

Shringar, or adornment, was considered almost a ritual for a bride. Traditionally and even today, at Hindu marriages the bride receive a beauty box from her husband. Today, synthetic mass manufactured vanity cases have replaced the ancient, adorably carved wooden chests or metal cases, once used by brides. Even the contents are mass products: a cream, a lipstick, a powder, and eyeliner and so on...as much as the purse permits. But in ancient times, the beauty box itself was a work of art. Much care was put into it and it was filled with all possible items for a woman's personal adornment. Glass or carved bottles of *attar* (extracts or perfumes) of roses, jasmine, mogra and many other flowers,

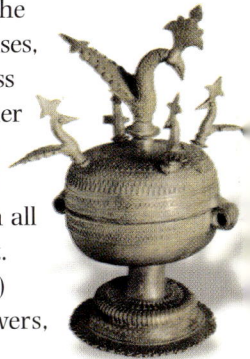

containers of kohl for the eyes, others even more intricately carved or shaped containing *abeer* (powder) or *missi* (a herb) to redden the lips were lovingly put into the make-up chest.

Today women all over the world are using henna to disguise white hair and turn it to a reddish brown shade. In ancient times henna has been used not only to enliven the hair but also to adorn the palms of the hands and feet and even colour the nails.

Teenagers today, eagerly buy the latest anti-acne and anti-pimple creams at exorbitant prices, little realising that the cure for these ills exists in their own kitchens! Women in India have used sandalwood for centuries for this very purpose. It has strong antiseptic qualities and softens the skin. Similarly, women in most eastern countries have used "chikni mitti" or Fuller's earth, mixed with rose water. This is also popularly known as "Cleopatra's Pack" in the west. It helps to tighten the skin, and is the basis on which facemasks are marketed.

Women in ancient times were very particular about removing unwanted hair. Thus ash from incense sticks was used to get rid of them. Lemon juice and sugar mix was also used regularly for this purpose. Today, women go to beauty parlors for "waxing". Nothing changes. The future goes way back. Centuries back.

Women in India have always used herbs, fruits and flowers to beautify themselves, to adorn and enhance their good points. We do indeed have a wealth of knowledge as far as herbal and natural beauty aids are

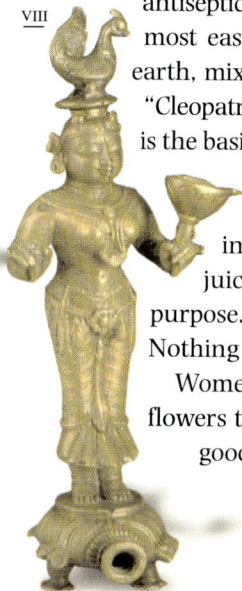

VIII

concerned. In fact beauty and make-up ritual in ancient times was more elaborate and state of the art than even today.

Exquisitely designed boxes and containers were used to store beauty aids. Historic evidence reveals that there was an intense desire for personal culture and body care. For instance, hair-drying pins of metal with intricately carved bases having devices for creating rhythmic sounds were used while drying the hair. These were very popular in South India. Among other objects of ancient toiletry articles, one can find slender bottles carved with tiny mirrors. *Kankavatis* were containers for a certain red pigment, used as bindis to mark the forehead. These containers had different forms like peacocks, musical instruments, elephants, swans, or were mango shaped.

Even the foot scrubbers found among ancient objects were imaginatively made. These also had a hollow shape and were fitted with tiny metal balls that made a rhythmic sound when used. Some other exquisitely shaped were containers for *Missi*, a herb to redden the lips; others contained different dyes to adorn the forehead. Carved boxes containing *Abeer* were also included. Abeer is a powder made from sandalwood, aloe, rose petals and a few grains of civet. These were powdered in a mortar to a very fine powder.

Thus the ancient art of makeup and adornment finds no comparison today. In this jet age of instant cures, we look backwards to the glorious days when it was difficult to find an ordinary face, when women made it a point to look extraordinary.

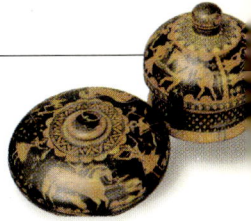

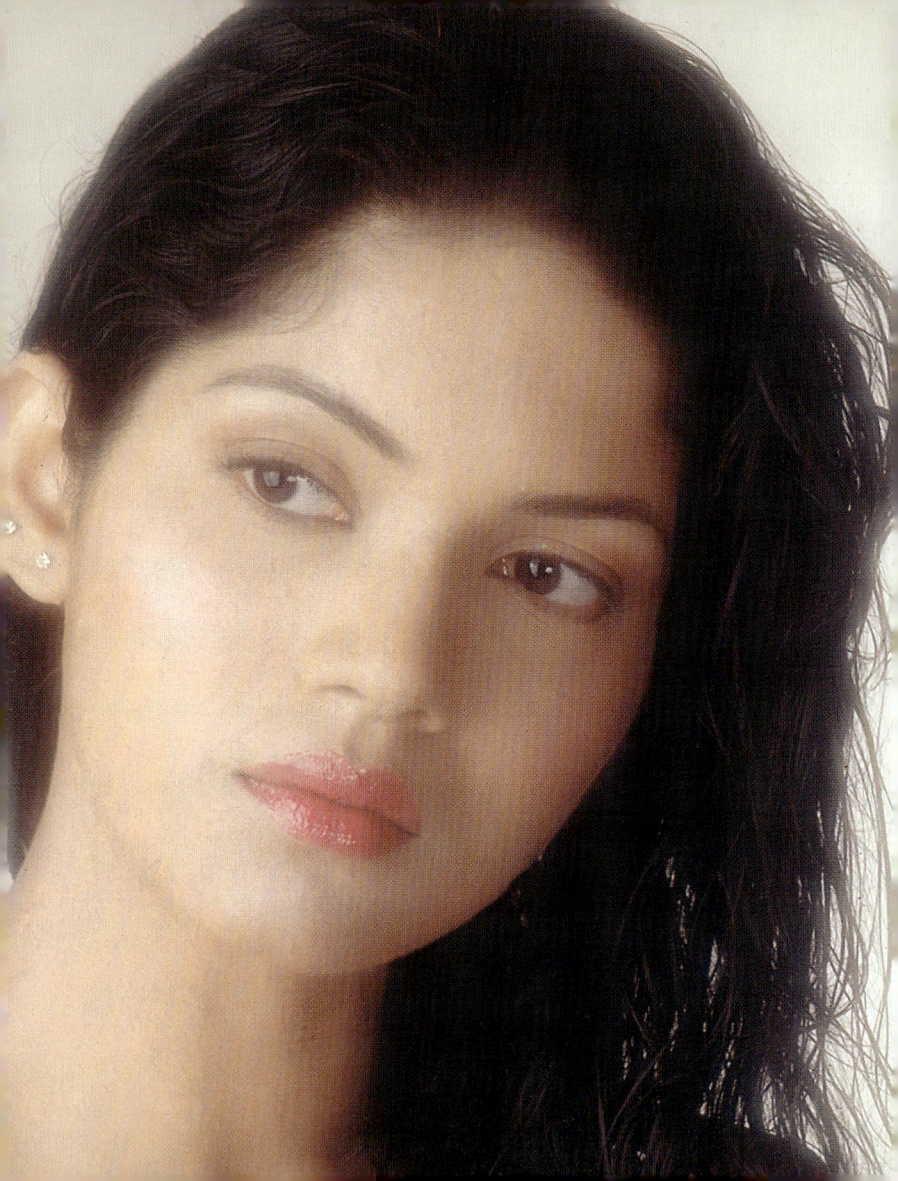

Your Face
Reflects Your Aura

Oriental women as well as those from Egypt, Rome and other ancient civilizations were known for their tremendous skills in beauty care. As the Italian writer Sonnini says about oriental women, in his book *Travels*: "Nowhere are the women more beautiful, nowhere are they better skilled or more practiced in the art of arresting or repairing the ravages of time." Indeed, oriental women have always exuded an aura of beauty. The aura of your personality is directly reflected on your face. It is one of the most expressive and delicate part of your body — it also bears the onslaught of age and weather more than any other part of the body. It therefore needs to be preserved and protected most preciously.

A beautiful face can be described as one which is cared for and which awakens admiration for that reason. From the earliest civilizations, women have searched for and used beauty cures and aids. Today, perfectly generated beauty cures are available and beauty culture is an enormous business, as can be seen from vast advertising budgets. Launches of beauty products are done on a very lavish scale. All kinds of incentives are offered to lure women to a product. Whenever women flip through a magazine, watch films or ramp shows, they wish that they too had the perfectly

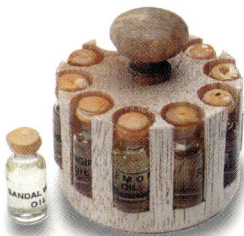

sculpted body and flawless skin like the models they see. Few women however realise that what they see is a perfectly "made-up" face and not necessarily a flawless beauty. Care for your skin can enable you to look beautiful. To make your face have the ability to "launch a thousand ships" and to acquire a beautiful and blemish-free skin, you need to pamper it.

"Back to nature" is the global mantra of beauty care today. You can enhance your beauty with the help of products provided by nature itself.

In ancient times too beauty care stemmed from nature, Perfumes made from flowers, barks of scented wood were mixed with oils and left to mature. Once the oils and the wood absorbed the fragrance of these flowers, they were converted to perfumes and scented oils for the body and face. These were lavishly used to prevent the skin from drying, and to protect it from the harsh elements of nature.

Women and men too, extensively used make-up in ancient times. Eye paint made from green malachite, grey ore, and galena was ground to a powder and mixed with oil to form kohl for the eyes. Various other cosmetics were made using nature's unlimited bounty.

Colour for lips, cheeks and nails was made from red ochre clay. Powders for whitening the face were used by Assyrian women even as long back as in 1000 BC. Special make-up jars, beautifully carved bottles made from stone and glass were used to store cosmetics. Thus, women in ancient times managed to

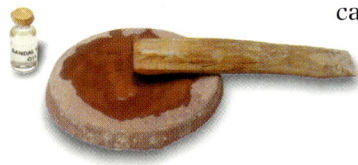

look stunning without using any chemical-based or synthetic cosmetics which did not exist then and yet their beauty had the power to bewitch.

Over the years, man developed mass-produced, synthetic beauty products. Contrary to their purpose, these have sometimes caused more problems than what they set out to cure. In fact, many doctors and cosmetologists believe that a number of skin problems can be attributed to synthetic beauty products. As a result, people are again moving towards natural beauty aids. Eco-friendly, natural cosmetics and beauty products are now in great demand. These truly enhance the quality of your skin and so make you look and feel healthier and lovelier.

Nature's bounty has provided us with a treasure chest, which if used effectively can bring out that special glow in your face. It is not necessary to spend a fortune to look beautiful. You can work wonders by just delving into your home's treasure trove of fruits, flowers, vegetables and condiments to find the right cure.

You must also accept yourself and turn your so-called "flaws" into features of your personality. For instance, a sharp pointed nose, or freckles or a mole on your cheek need not be camouflaged; any or all of these can become a distinctive part of your personality, to be used as an advantage. Besides, most common problems can be cured at home. Do you have under-eye shadows? Are you worried about wrinkles? What about pimples? Head towards the kitchen and help yourself to its bounty, which if used the right way could well be that Alladin's lamp which lights up your beautiful face.

Skin Problems
Facial Facts

Some of the most common problems that women have are related to the skin. Freckles, dry skin, wrinkles, pimples and oily skin, shadows — the list is endless. A little knowledge of their causes and prevention can go a long way in combating them. Some problems are genetic while others are merely a part of the ageing process. Today, women face a host of hair and skin problems. This is mainly due to poor food habits, a disorganised lifestyle and of course, environmental pollution. Here we would like to deal with some of these problems and suggest some really wonderful home cures for them.

Today, international beauty houses are being compelled to use natural products as the modern, health and beauty conscious woman is going back to nature. These cures yield better and longer lasting results. They enhance the beauty of your face and radiate that special aura from within you.

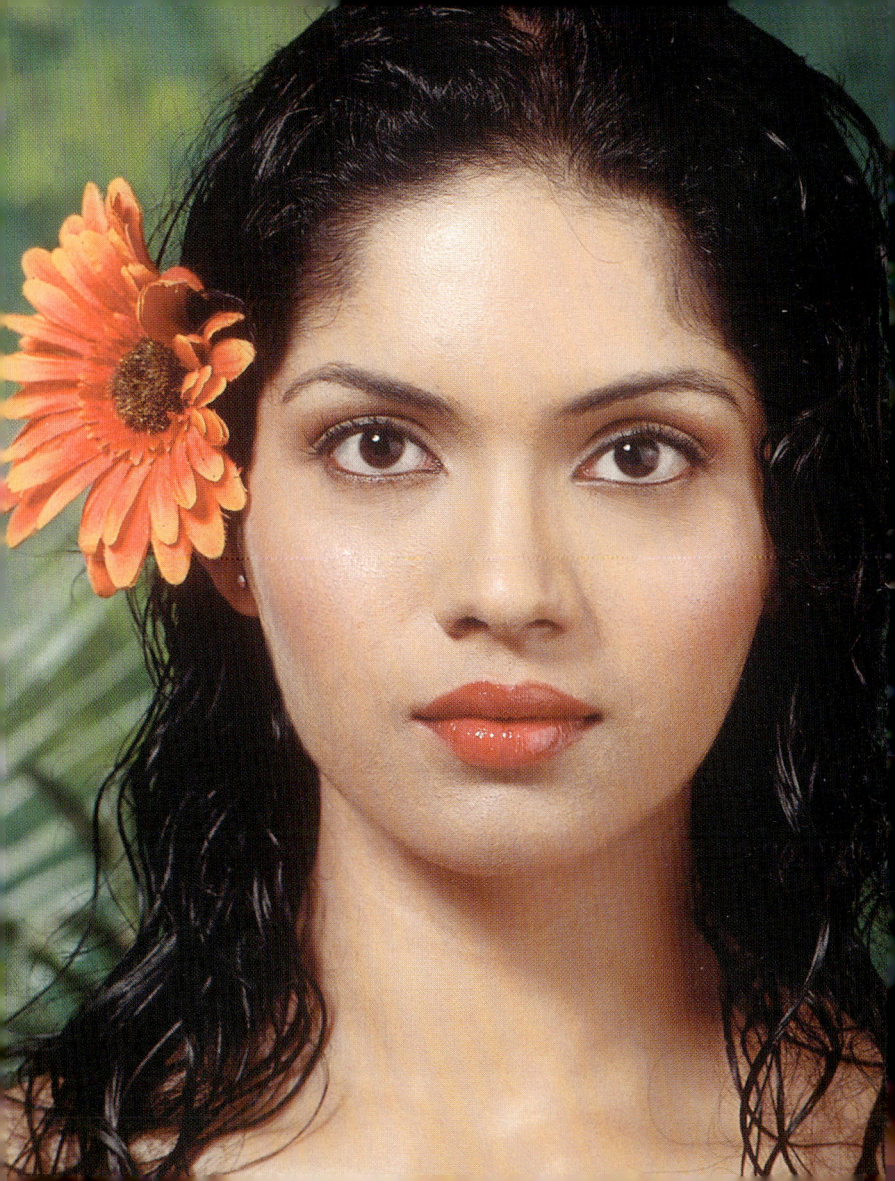

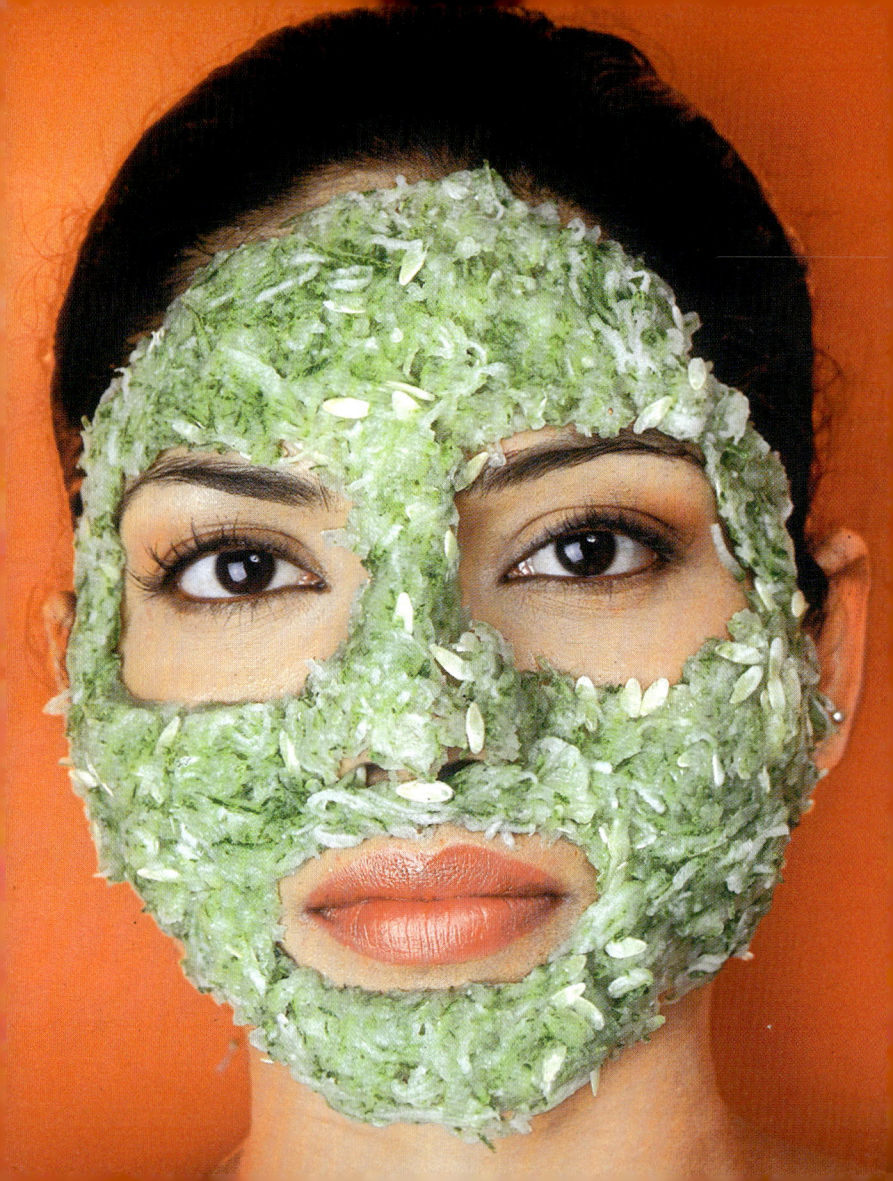

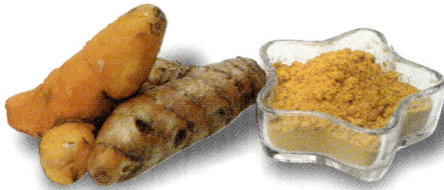

Cleansers

Face care begins with a good wash. Cleansing creams and lotions are used to remove stale make-up and dirt. If this is not regularly done, then the pores get clogged leading to numerous skin problems. Here are some easy to make, and even easier to use, face cleansers suitable for different types of skin.

CHICKPEA POWDER AND TURMERIC: Take half cup chickpea powder. Add one teaspoon turmeric powder and half cup of milk. Stir well. Apply this paste all over the forehead, face and neck. Wait for two minutes and wash off. This is good for oily or mixed skin types. The chickpea powder absorbs the extra oil and the milk nourishes your skin, leaving it tingling fresh.

MILK: Nature's most effective natural cleanser. Take half a cup of cold milk. Add half teaspoon of salt. Stir. Take balls of cotton, soak and then gently dab milk and salt lotion all over forehead, face, and neck. Leave it on for 2-3 minutes. Apply again. Now rub gently in circular motions and wash off. The salt in the milk gently exfoliates dead skin and the milk nourishes the skin. Your face instantly

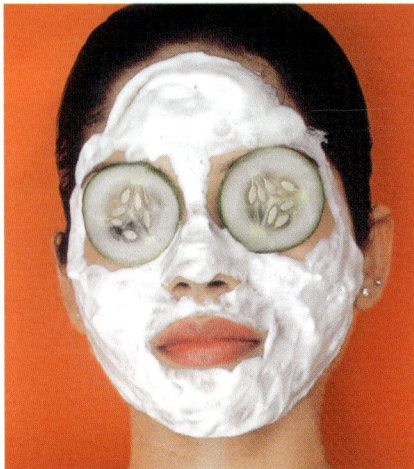

gets a fresh and glowing look. This is good for all skin types.

CUCUMBER AND CURD: Take one cucumber, grate it. Squeeze out the juice. Add to this 3-4 tablespoons of beaten curds. Stir well. Apply this paste all over the forehead, face and neck. Leave it on for 3-4 minutes. Wash face and neck with cold water. While cleaning and tightening the pores, it also lightens blemishes and freckles. Very nourishing for the skin. You could use just grated cucumber as a face cleanser too.

YOGHURT: This is yet another effective face cleanser, very good for dry skin. Take half a cup yoghurt. Add to this half teaspoon honey. Stir well. Apply all over the forehead, face and neck. Rub it in gently. Leave on for 2-3 minutes. Wash off with cold water.

CHAMOMILE: Take a handful of fresh chamomile flowers. Add to these some rosemary tops, fresh or dry. Boil them well in a pan containing 2 cups of water. Let the mixture cool. Mash flowers well. Strain and keep. When cool, dip in small pieces of muslin, wring and apply all over the forehead, face and neck. Keep dipping and applying several times. Let it dry. Wash off when completely dry. An excellent cleanser.

ALMOND: Take 5-7 almonds. Pound them to a paste/powder. Take the yolk of one egg. Beat it up. Add to it one tablespoon of honey and continue beating. Now add almond paste/powder. Mix well. Apply all over the forehead, face and neck. Rub it in gently. When it begins to dry, wash off with lukewarm water. Good for dry skins, especially in winter when the skin tends to lose its natural oils. This acts as a restorative.

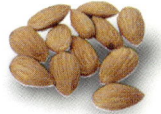

9

HONEY AND VITAMIN A/E: This is a very good and effective cleanser, especially for people with blemishes. Take half cup warm water. Add one-tablespoon honey. Snip open one capsule of vitamin A and one capsule of vitamin E. Mix well. Apply quickly all over the face. Leave it on for 2 minutes and wash with cold water.

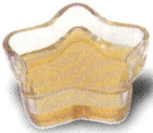

These cleansers can be used in the mornings before a bath, however, it is imperative to use them at bedtime. Remove all traces of make-up with milk, or rosewater and glycerine cleansers everyday, and use any of the others occasionally to treat your skin to a special cleansing routine.

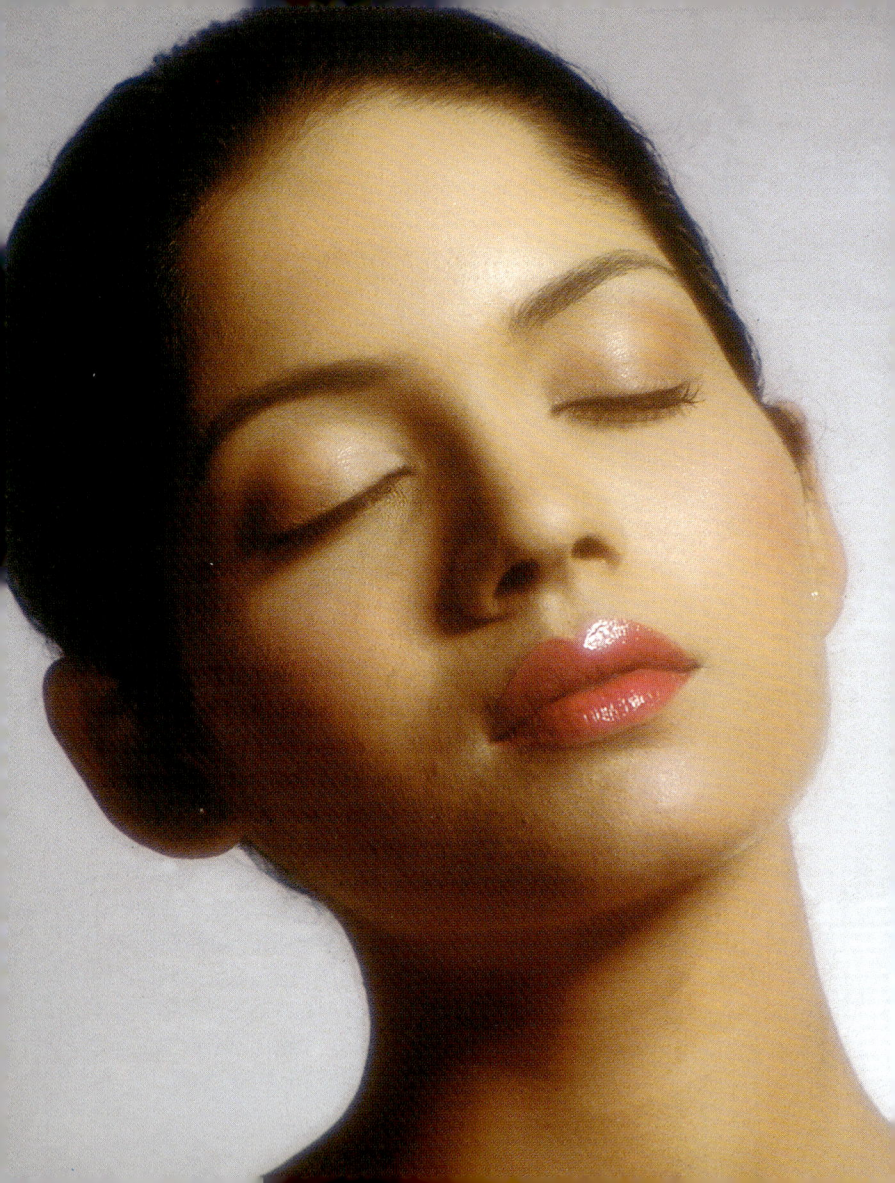

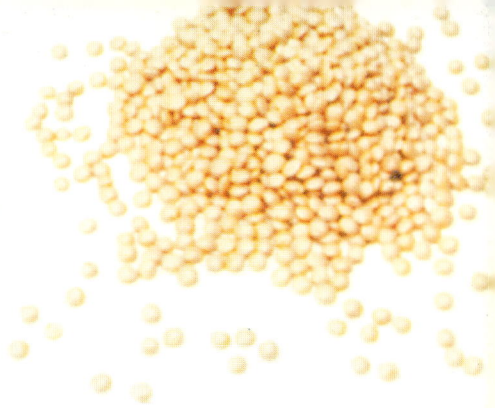

Rejuvenate with Exfoliates

Sometimes one needs a more exhaustive cleansing routine. These need not be a daily ritual, but they are required to rejuvenate your skin, more so, if one has skin problems. You also need to get rid of dead skin cells. For this you need to use exfoliates.

True, exfoliation is great as it stimulates the skin, and helps to get rid of dead skin cells leading to a clearer skin with fewer lines and wrinkles. A word of caution here, everything is good within limits. Many women believe that they should exfoliate everyday. Be cautious. One should never over-exfoliate as that may damage blood vessels especially the delicate skin area on the face. This can cause redness and inflammation. Your skin type determines how often you should exfoliate. Ideally speaking, it should be done once a week. Women who have abnormally oily skins and an acne problem can do so twice a week. Never more than that. In winters, exfoliate less often than in summers.

Basically there are two types of exfoliates — mechanical and chemical. Mechanical exfoliates involve using an abrasive sponge or loofah to physically buff the skin. Sometimes using these too harshly can harm your skin. Instead, you could use mechanical exfoliates made from grains, pulses or even vegetables. Chemical exfoliates are commercially marketed products which use beta hydroxy acids to remove dead skin cells. These should be used only when advised by a beautician or cosmetologist. For normal requirements it is best to use exfoliates made from natural substances.

OATMEAL: Take half cup oatmeal. Add to this half teaspoon salt, one teaspoon honey and just a little cold milk to make a rough thick paste. Apply all over the forehead, face and neck. When it begins to dry up, rub using brisk, firm movements. A good exfoliate for tough skins acts as an abrasive agent and helps in exfoliation.

WHEAT HUSK: The flaky powder left behind when wheat flour is made, is the best exfoliate. You could use wheat porridge grains also. Take half cup of wheat husk or porridge. Add to this one tablespoon honey and one tablespoon of milk. Make a thick paste. Apply all over the forehead, face and neck (avoid the eyes). Exfoliate gently with a loofah, or use strong circular motions with the hand, keep rubbing for 5 minutes. Wash off. The skin is clean, baby soft and glowing.

CHICKPEA POWDER: Take half cup chickpea powder. Add one teaspoon turmeric powder and one tablespoon olive oil (or any

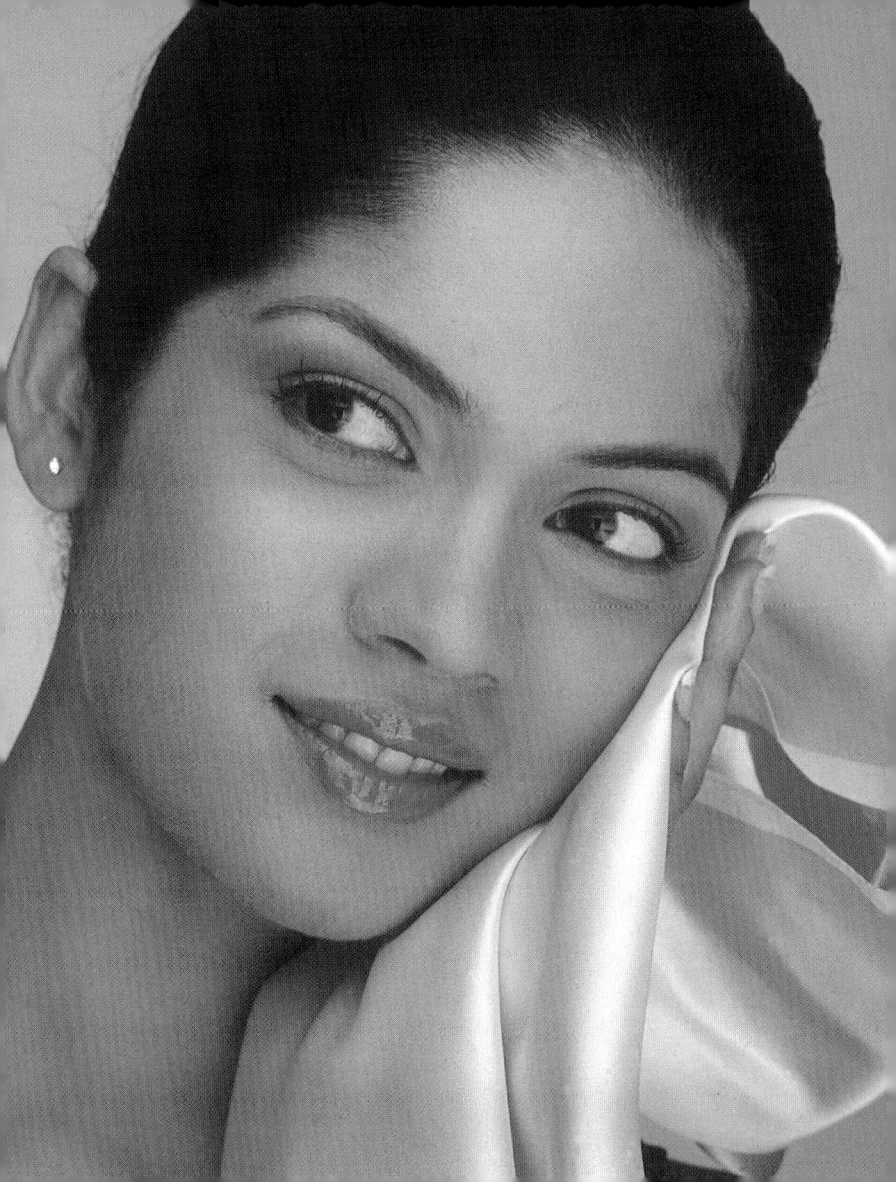

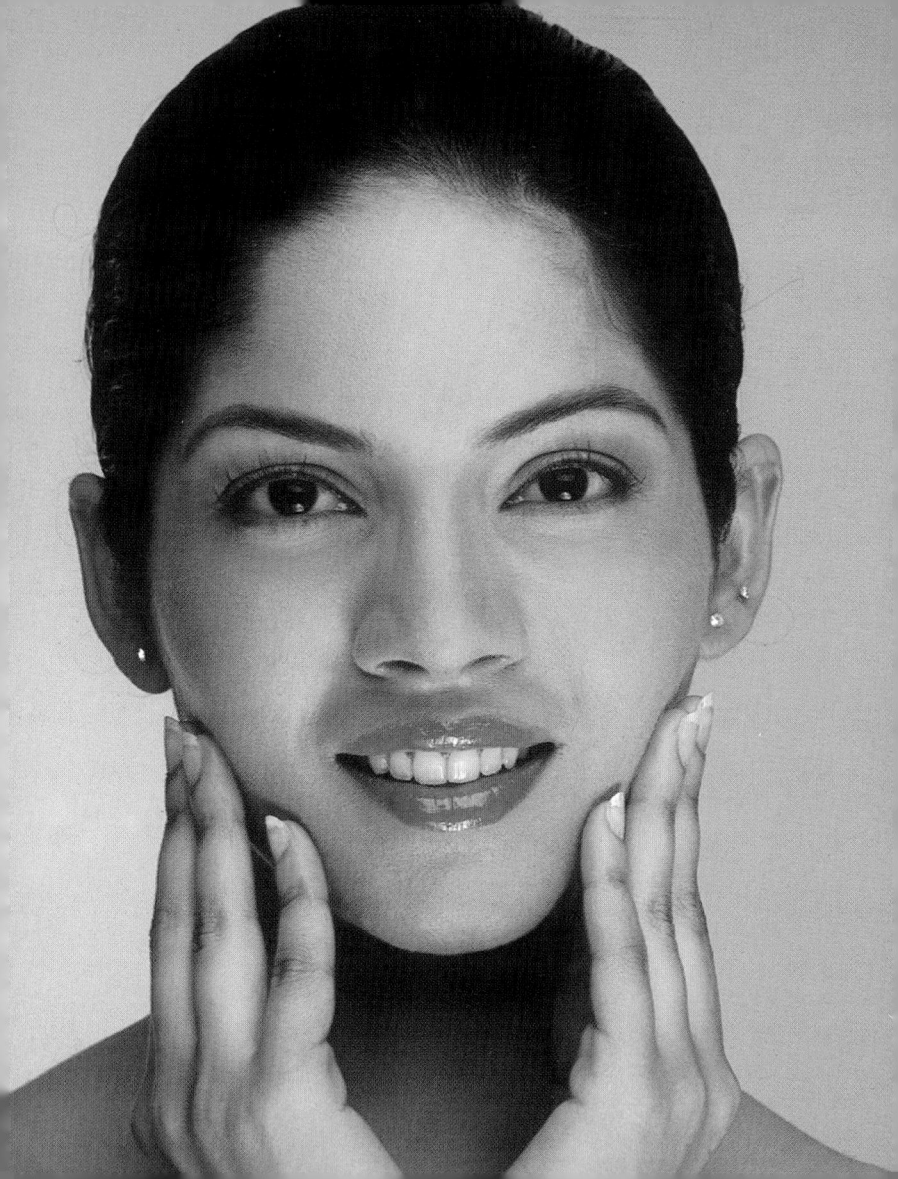

other oil like coconut). Mix and make a thick paste. Apply all over the forehead, face and neck (avoid the eyes).

When the paste starts to dry up, rub with your hands, scrubbing as you go along. Then wash it off with lukewarm water. This is a mild but effective exfoliate that also helps get rid of fine facial hair.

RICE: This makes an excellent exfoliate. Take half cup rice. Grind it coarsely to a powder. Add to it one tablespoon of honey and two tablespoons of beaten curds. Blend into a paste. Apply all over the forehead, face and neck. This paste dries up very fast, so rub quickly in circular motions. Scrub well and wash off.

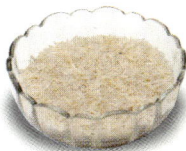

15

YELLOW LENTIL: Take half cup of any yellow lentil. Soak for half an hour. Drain out the water. Coarse grind it to a paste. Add to it a tablespoon of chickpea powder with just enough milk to make a thick paste. Apply all over the forehead, face and neck. Keep rubbing in circular motions to remove dead skin and clear blemishes. This is an ideal exfoliate for even very tender skin.

VEGETABLES: You can use cabbage leaves, the outer skin of sweet gourd, skin of tomato etc. Take grated cabbage leaves, tied in a thin piece of muslin and rub all over the forehead, face and neck. Keep rubbing, applying pressure. The same can be done with any other vegetable peels, or grated sweet gourd. These are the mildest of exfoliates and clean very gently.

Toners and Fresheners

Toners, fresheners and astringents belong to the same family. They help in smoothening your skin, and act as a balm after the exfoliation process. These help to seal skin pores, tighten the outer layers of the facial skin, also acting as a safety net after a heavy exfoliation and cleansing routine.

BERRIES: You could use strawberries, cherries, cranberries or blackberries to make this unique, rejuvenating toner and astringent at home.

Take one tablespoon honey, 2 tablespoons of pureed berries, one tablespoon oatmeal or wheat bran. Combine all the ingredients in a bowl. Wet your face. Apply this paste all over the forehead, face and neck (avoid the eyes). Let it remain for five minutes. Now gently rub it into your face. Rub and wash off with tepid water. The fruit acids in the berries shrink your pores, brighten up your face and tone your skin. Use this toner to really pamper yourself.

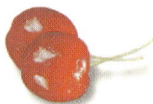

LIME: Take 2 cups of water. Add juice of two limes. To this solution add one tablespoon of tincture of benzoin as a preservative. Shake well and pour into a bottle and keep. Use this as an astringent. Very good for normal skin.

WATERCRESS: Take a handful of watercress salad leaves. Bruise them and add them to a saucepan containing equal parts of

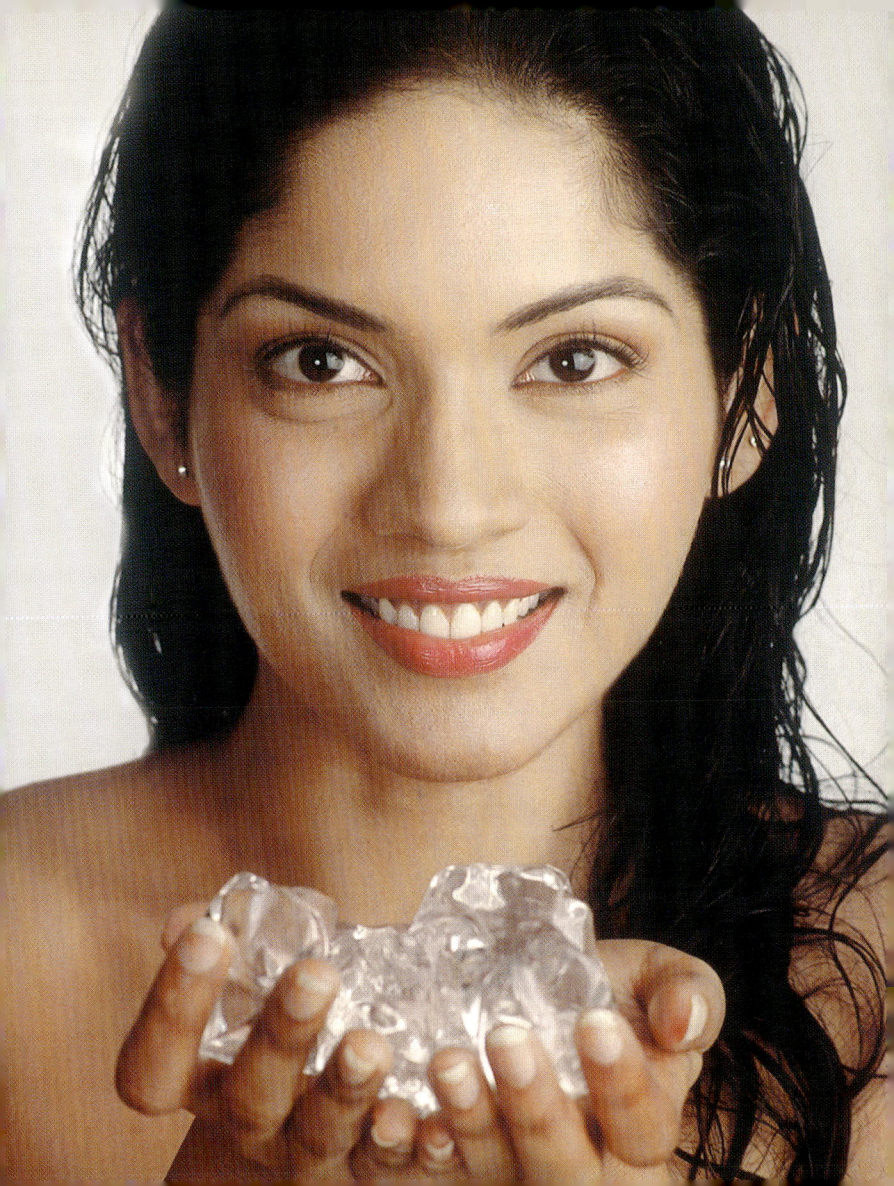

water and milk (one and a half cups should be enough). Simmer over a slow fire for a few minutes. Remove from the fire and mash the leaves well. Strain and pour the liquid into a bottle after cooling. Apply this lotion after a bath or after cleaning your face of all make-up. Let it dry on your face. This removes blemishes and gives the complexion a healing touch, making it soft and creamy. Wash off after 10-15 minutes.

CORNFLOWER: Take a handful of flowers and infuse in 250 ml of boiling water. Allow to cool. Mash the steamed flowers into the water. Add a teaspoon of witch hazel (available at the chemist shop). Strain and pour into a bottle after cooling. An effective and soothing astringent.

ORANGE AND LEMON PEELS: Do not throw away orange and lemon peels. Sun dry them. When they are absolutely dry and brittle, powder them and keep them in a jar or wide mouthed bottle. This powder can be used in a number of face care preparations; as a moisturizing face pack, as an exfoliate and also as an astringent.

To use as an astringent, take 2 tablespoons of this powder, add to this 3 tablespoons of rosewater and 3 tablespoons of water. Stir well and shake it up. Apply this lotion all over the forehead, face and neck. Be careful and avoid the eyes. Let it dry, then wash off. This is an excellent

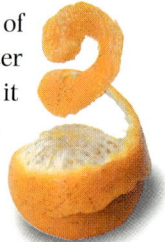

astringent that cures blemishes, shrinks open pores and is a good cure for pimples.

CUCUMBER AND ROSEWATER: Take one cucumber. Peel and grate it. Take 3 tablespoons of rosewater and add the grated cucumber. Put it in a blender and make a paste and refrigerate. Use as a toner on dry sun-burnt skin. Apply all over; leave it on for 20 minutes. Rinse off. Excellent for sun burnt, dry skin.

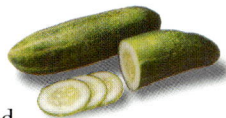

ICE CUBES: Take ice cubes and rub them all over the face. This tightens the pores and increases the blood circulation. An ideal, inexpensive and instant toner.

LEMON TREE FLOWERS: If you have a lime tree in your garden, you can make this effective complexion lotion. Take a handful of lemon flowers and infuse them in 250 ml of boiling water. Let it cool. Mash flowers and strain. To this add equal part of rose water. Pour in a bottle, refrigerate and keep. Use after a bath or after cleaning your face. Especially good after you apply at bedtime and leave it on overnight.

Moisturisers and Face Packs

A rigorous cleaning and exfoliating routine leaves the skin hungry for food and nourishment. You need a good moisturiser or face pack to nourish your skin. In fact you need to use moisturisers at least twice a day. Moisturisers nourish the skin, making it supple and soft.

EGG AND ALMOND MOISTURISER: Take one egg yolk and add to it one tablespoon almond oil or take 5 almonds and crush them to a fine powder and then add to the egg yolk. Add one tablespoon of honey to this. Stir well and apply to the forehead, face and neck (avoid the eyes). Leave it on for 15 minutes. Rinse, first with warm water then with cold.

FULLER'S EARTH AND HONEY: Take 2 tablespoons of fuller's earth. Add to it one tablespoon of honey and one tablespoon of milk. Mix well. Apply this paste all over the forehead, face and neck (avoid the eyes). Leave it on for 15 minutes, and then wash off with cold water. The fuller's earth seals the pores while the honey and milk nourish the skin.

MARIGOLD FLOWERS: Take 2 cups of marigold petals. Soak them in a bowl of water and keep aside. After 2-3 hours, when the petals are limp, mash them well with your hands in the same water. To this paste add one tablespoon of glycerine. Mix well. Apply to the forehead, face and neck (avoid the eyes). Wash off

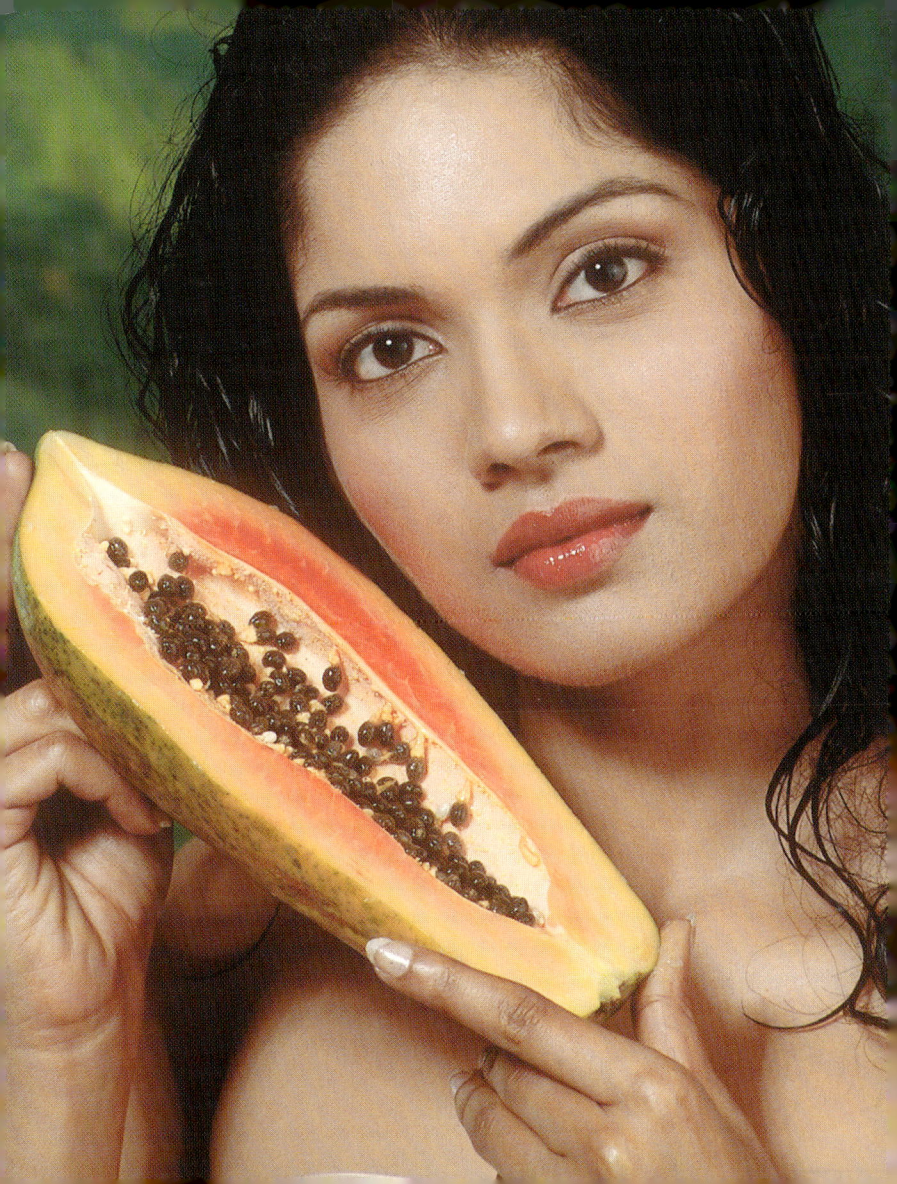

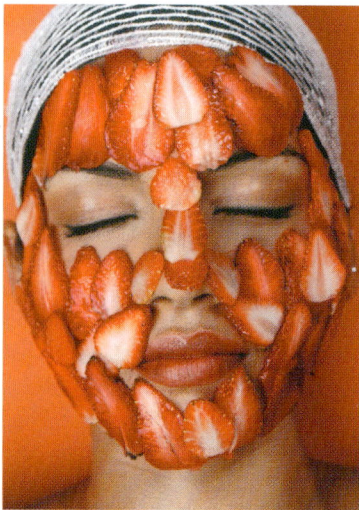

after 10 minutes. An unusual, but very effective, skin tonic.

STRAWBERRIES: An excellent nourishment for people with oily skin. It feeds your skin yet, absorbs excess oil. Take a handful of strawberries, chop and put in blender. Add the juice of one lime and half cup yoghurt or cream and blend well. Pour in a container, refrigerate for 30 minutes and apply to the forehead, face and neck (avoid the eyes). When it begins to cake, apply again. Let it stand for 20 minutes, then rinse off by rubbing gently into the skin.

LEMON JELLY: Take a packet of lemon jelly and add to it a cup of boiling water. Stir and mix well, and add to this the juice of one lemon. Stir and let it set in the refrigerator. Just before using, steam your face to open up the pores. Apply chilled jelly to the forehead, face and neck (avoid the eyes). Leave it on for 15 minutes then rinse off. This is an excellent cure for oily skin as lemon absorbs the excess oil from your skin.

PARSLEY: Take a handful of parsley. Chop it finely and put it in a bowl. Pour 2-3 tablespoons of boiling water over it. Add one tablespoon of light olive oil and mash well to make a thick paste. Apply to the forehead, face and neck (avoid the eyes). Leave it on for 5-10 minutes. Remove gently. Wash it off with warm water. Parsley has antibiotic properties that kills germs. The olive oil helps to shrink the pores. This pack is especially useful when you come back from a polluted environment. Useful for all skin types.

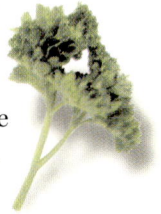

WATERMELON: There is no better method of refreshing the body and sun-scorched face than to use a watermelon. Watermelon instantly restores lost moisture, tightens the skin and leaves it looking fresh. It is also simple to use. Just cut slices of watermelon, squeeze some lime juice on them and apply to the forehead, face and neck (avoid the eyes). Keep rubbing in hard circular motions as you go along. Alternatively, you could puree the fruit, add lime juice and apply like a face pack. Leave it on for 20 minutes and wash it off. A squeaky clean, glowing skin emerges.

AVOCADO: Very popular with most beauticians, who make liberal use of this fruit for a variety of beauty treatments. Chop and put the fruit in a blender. Add one teaspoon honey, a little lemon juice and half cup yoghurt. Blend to make a thick paste.

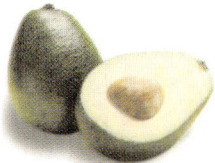

Pour into a jar and refrigerate for 30 minutes. Massage well into the face and neck. Wash off with plain water.

APRICOT: Another favourite with beauticians, also used in several beauty care products too. Take 2-3 apricots, de-seed them, chop and put them in a blender. Add to this half cup yoghurt or thick cream. Whip and pour into a container. Apply to the forehead, face and neck (avoid the eyes). When it starts caking, apply some more. Let it stand for 20 minutes, then wash off. It's an excellent nourishment for your skin.

PAPAYA: You can use the papaya fruit instead of the apricot to make a similar skin nourishment potion. Papaya effectively rejuvenates tired, jaded and dry skin. Regular use yields astonishing results.

ALMOND: Take 10-15 almonds and grind them finely. Take half cupful of yoghurt or sour cream. Add to it the almond powder and mix well to form a smooth paste. Apply to the forehead, face and neck (avoid the eyes). Leave it on for 20 minutes and then wash off. An excellent tonic for dry blemished skin.

OATS: Take a cupful of oatmeal. Add beaten yolks of 2 eggs and one tablespoon of honey. Add a few drops of tincture of benzoin. Whip all this together in a bowl. Pour in a jar and keep in the refrigerator. You can use this several times. Take a little of this thick creamy paste and apply to the forehead, face and neck (avoid the eyes). Massage into the skin and leave it on for 15 minutes. Rinse off with lukewarm water.

ORANGE PEEL AND ROSEWATER: Take 3 tablespoons of dry orange peel powder and add to this a few dried powdered rose petals. Add one teaspoon of honey and just enough milk to form a thick paste. Apply to the forehead, face and neck (avoid the eyes). Let it stand for 20 minutes, then wash off. This unique moisturising pack leaves your skin as soft as a baby's skin.

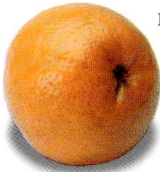

25

You can certainly arrest ageing and keep your skin looking healthy by following these simple, yet, very effective face-care rituals and routines. This does not mean that there are no other skin problems that have to be dealt with. Pimples, pigmentation, dry skin, wrinkles, oily skin and blackheads are some of the common problems that women face. Given here are a few simple, easy to make cures for some. Patience is the keyword for effective treatment; the results will far exceed your expectations.

Growing Up With Acne

Every age has its own problems. Acne, pimples and blackheads are some of the common problems that cause anguish during the process of growing up.

Yes, it is mostly a problem with adolescents, though it could be due to hormonal imbalance too. The female hormones, estrogen and progesterone are produced during the early growing up years, and the body needs time to adjust to this. An imbalance is created. The androgen hormones produced by the adrenal glands also affect the texture of the skin. The result of all these hormonal changes can manifest into excessive oiliness of the skin and scalp and also excessive perspiration. Too much secretion of oil clogs the pores, leading to blackheads and spots. Infected blackheads may lead to acne and pimples. A very aggressive cleanliness regime is needed to combat this situation. A few simple Do's and Don'ts will help.

Don't ever "pick" a pimple. The natural healing cycle for a pimple is 7 days. According to dermatologists, when you "pick" a pimple, you interrupt this cycle and set back the healing process by another 7 days. The best thing is to sit on and let it dry on its own.

DO'S
- Drink lots of water.
- Clean your face as often as you can.
- Use astringents to help get rid of excess oil.
- Eat more fruits and raw vegetables.

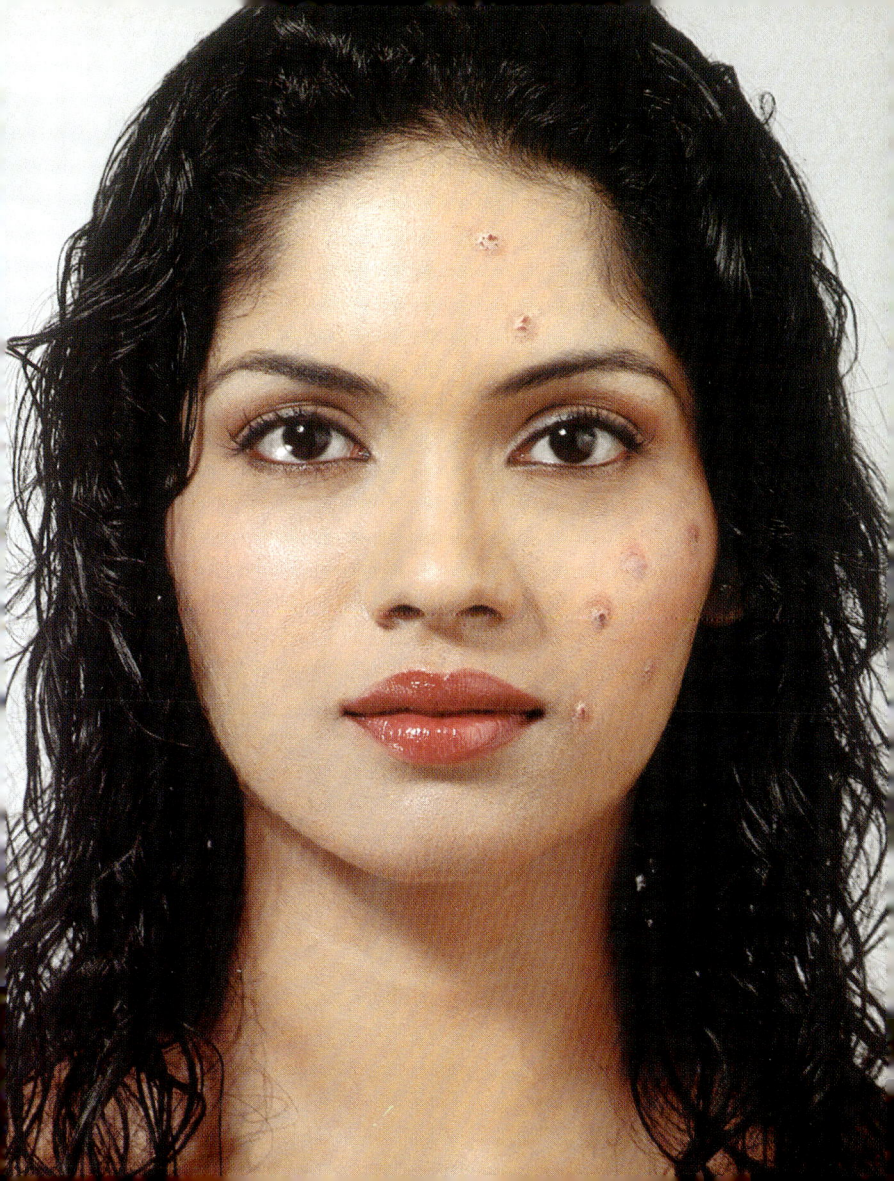

● Bathe frequently and use cooling lotions during summer.
● Keep your nails trimmed neatly to avoid dirt being carried to your face and increase chances of infection.

DON'T
● Eat oily and starchy foods.
● Use any make-up.

Blackheads, acne and pimples can indeed be controlled with the help of ingredients from your kitchen. A word of caution. If your infection is mild, then these simple remedies along with a controlled diet will suffice. However for major infections it is best to take the doctor's advice too.

BLACK PEPPER AND CURD: Take one tablespoon black pepper powder and add to it enough curd to make a thick paste. Apply on the infected area and let it dry. Wash off after 5-7 minutes. This is an effective cure for blackheads.

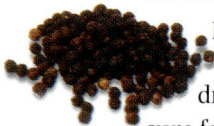

OATMEAL AND YOGHURT: Take 2 tablespoons of oatmeal and 3 tablespoons of yoghurt. Mix and add one tablespoon of lemon juice and one teaspoon of olive oil. Blend and whisk well together in a bowl. Wash your hands and then apply over infected area first, then all over the face. Leave on for 5-7 minutes and then rinse with cold water. Very effective for blackheads.

TOMATO JUICE: Normally, pimples and acne are associated with an oily skin. In case these occur on a dry skin then this is the ideal treatment. Take a few tomatoes and puree them. Freeze the puree into cubes (in an ice cube tray). Store these frozen tomato ice cubes in a bag or a container in the freezer. During the day, apply one cube each on either cheek, all the time rubbing gently. Repeat the treatment everyday. A very effective way of getting rid of pimples.

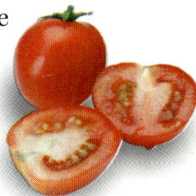

ALMOND, LEMON AND OLIVE OIL: Powder 10 almonds and add to this the juice of 2 lemons. Add 2 tablespoons of olive oil, mix well and store. Keep in a jar and use twice a day. Its helps in curing pimples.

POTATO AND MILK: Pimples leave behind an ugly scar when they dry and fall off. To get rid of these scars use this and see the results. Take 2 potatoes. Skin and grate them. Extract the juice and to this add 2-3 tablespoons of cold milk. Stir well and apply all over the pimple scars. Let it dry and gently rub and wash off. Use this treatment regularly, at least twice a day.

ORANGE PEEL AND YOGHURT: An ideal mask that extracts dirt and oil from clogged pores. It also opens up the clogged pores that cause acne and blackheads. Take 2 tablespoons of orange peel powder and add 4 tablespoons of yoghurt to make a paste. Apply

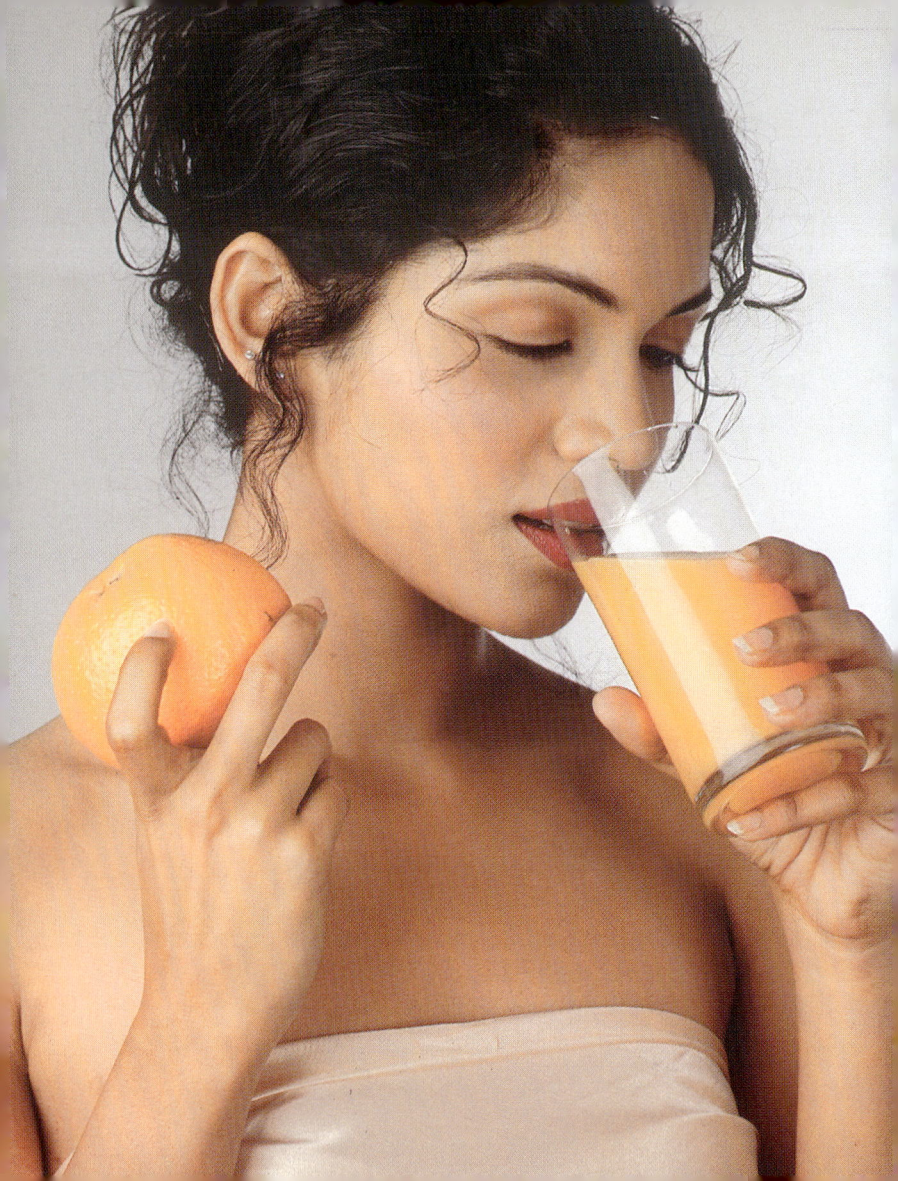

all over the face, while gently rubbing in circular motion. Wash off with cold water. An excellent way to prevent clogged pores and keep the skin clean and healthy.

APPLE JUICE: Take an apple, peel and grate it to extract the juice. Add one teaspoon of honey and apply on face. Dab gently on the pimples and let it dry. Apply again. Repeat this treatment at least twice a day. Your pimples will dry and the scars will vanish with regular treatment.

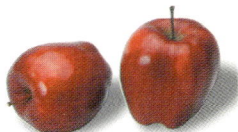

GARLIC: Take a few pods of garlic and crush them fine. Add a few drops of honey and add some curd to make a paste. Apply gently only on the pimples. Let it dry, and then wash gently without scrubbing. Regular use helps dry the pimples faster and healing is much quicker. Be careful to use this paste only on the pimples.

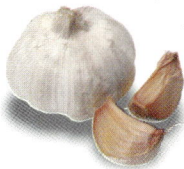

TOMATO AND YOGHURT: Take 2-3 tablespoons of tomato puree and add a little beaten yoghurt. Also add one tablespoon boiled oatmeal paste or boiled porridge. Blend all these into a paste. Apply all over the face and let it dry. Rinse with cold water. An effective way to rid yourself of pimples.

MINT: Take a few mint leaves and crush them finely. Tie them in a piece of muslin and squeeze it to extract the juice. Apply the juice all over the face. Dab gently with cotton wool pads on the pimples. Wash off and use at least once a week. It controls pimples.

FULLER'S EARTH AND ROSEWATER: This makes an ideal acne pack for oily skin. Take 2 tablespoons of fuller's earth and add one tablespoon of rosewater and 2 tablespoons of curd. Mix all these to form a thick paste. Apply this on the face and leave it for 20 minutes, and then wash it off. Regular use once a week is good for mild acne problems.

EAU DE COLOGNE AND LEMON JUICE: Mix an equal quantity of eau de cologne with boiled and cooled lemon juice. Apply this solution on the pimples. Leave to dry and then apply again. Wash off after the application has dried. Repeat the treatment at night. This helps in drying the pimples faster.

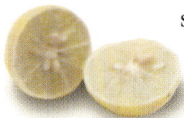

CLOVES: Take a few pods of cloves and roast them dry in a pan. Powder them and add a little curd to make a paste. Dab the paste on the pimples and let it dry. Wash off. Use this treatment regularly if you are prone to pimples. It is especially good for people who have an oily skin. The roasted cloves help to dry up the pimples faster.

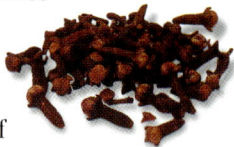

TEA BAGS: Saturate 2 tea bags in warm water. Now press the wet tea bags onto the pimples. Press, dab 2 or 3 times on pimples and leave it to dry. Rinse after a while.

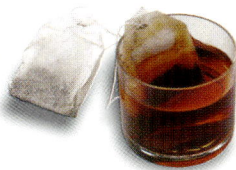

A few handy tips for those who suffer from pimple 'attacks'. Drink plenty of water and vegetable or fruit juices. Use cucumber or other fruit and vegetable packs to cure pimple scars. Maintain a diet that is rich in cottage cheese, fish and yoghurt. These help to cleanse your system and ward off pimples.

Every morning the first thing you should have is a glass of carrot juice or a glass of lime juice with honey. These are excellent 'tonics' to cleanse your system and help in giving you a clean, glowing complexion.

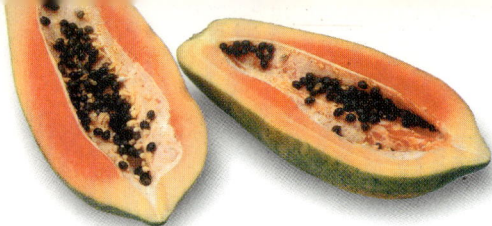

Blemishes, Shadows and Scars

Exposure to the sun and the vagaries of nature lead to different reactions on the skin. Some people get scars and blemishes while others suffer from sunburn and tan. A few precautionary measures and regular application of useful remedies would certainly help you combat these problems.

Stress levels generally alter the hormonal balance and this affects the appearance of your whole body. Further, pollution plays havoc on your skin. These are the two modern day culprits for most skin problems. Worry and sleeplessness cause shadows under the eyes; so does a faulty diet, smoking or inhalation of toxic fumes.

Shadows can also be due to an anaemic condition. Get your haemoglobin level checked. Have food that contain phosphorous, iron and proteins like bananas, plums and apples.

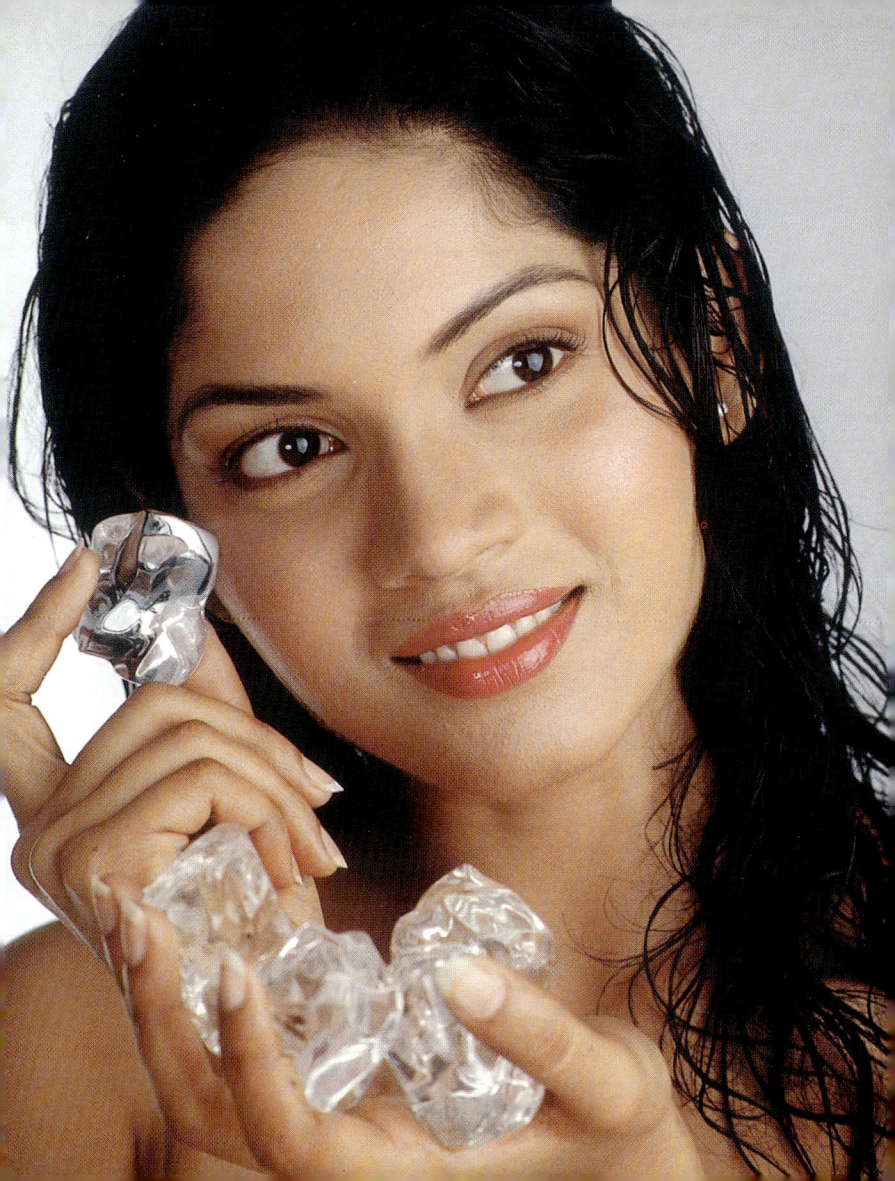

UNDER-EYE SHADOWS.

These are usually caused by tension and tiredness of the eyes. Overwork, long hours of exposure of work at a computer screen, lack of sleep and of course ageing process - all contribute to this problem. One tends to rush and buy the latest 'under-eye' cream. A word of caution here, some of them may be too rich and eztra moisturising and could result in causing puffiness in the under-eye area. Always use a light moisture-based cream. To cure these problems at home use the following:

CUCUMBER: Clean your face of all makeup. Cut out thin slices of cucumber. Chill them. Now lie down and shut your eyes. Apply chilled cucumber slices over your eyes and under-eye area and relax. Leave it on for 15 minutes. Gently rub the slices over the eyes and under-eye areas, and then wash off. You will feel relaxed and refreshed. The natural moisture from the cucumber acts as a healing tonic, while the cucumber juice helps to lighten the skin too. A great relief for tired and puffy eyes.

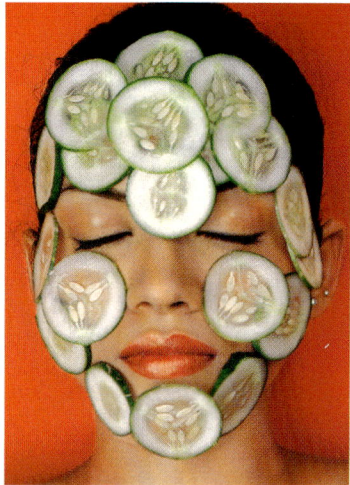

ICE CUBES: When you get in from the hot sun your eyes get tired and bloodshot. You also develop dark circles and shadows due to the heat and pollution. Try this: wash your face. Take some ice cubes and wrap them in two pieces of muslin. Lie down and shut your eyes. Place one ice cube pack over each eye, rubbing gently. This will immediately ease the 'burnt up skin' feeling. Regular use helps to lighten the shadows under the eyes.

GREEN GOURD: You could similarly use slices of green gourd instead of cucumber. The juice of the green gourd also helps in lightly moisturizing as well as lightening the skin tones.

PATCHES ON THE FACE

Sometimes due to hormonal changes, lack of proper nourishment or even due to stress, your facial skin becomes patchy— light in certain areas and dark in others. Use the following to get rid of patches as well as shadows and 'brown' spots.

FULLER'S EARTH AND LIME: Take one tablespoon fuller's earth, add one teaspoon of lime juice and enough rosewater to make a smooth paste. Apply this paste all over the face, rubbing it in gently. Leave it to dry and then apply again on the dark patches or spots. Leave it on for a further 5-7 minutes then wash and rinse with cold water. Use this treatment everyday to get rid of the patches.

MINT JUICE: Take a few mint leaves and crush them. Tie in a piece of muslin and extract its juice. Use this pure mint juice all over the face. Excellent for spots and blemishes.

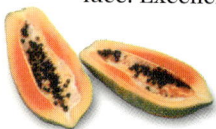

PAPAYA PACK: Take 2-3 slices of a ripe papaya and extract the pulp. Add to it one teaspoon of turmeric powder and one tablespoon of fuller's earth. Mash together to form a paste. Apply generously on the patches and dark areas of the skin. Leave it to dry. Then rinse it off. Regular use, maybe three times a week helps to even out the patches and blemishes.

CUCUMBER AND LIME JUICE: Take a cucumber and grate it after peeling. To this add juice of one lime. Mix well and put it into a blender to make a fine paste. Apply this paste all over the face and let it dry. Wash off. Regular use lightens shadows and scars.

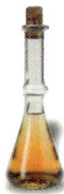

VINEGAR AND ROSEWATER: Take 2 tablespoons of vinegar and add one tablespoon of rosewater. Now add the juice of one cucumber. Stir well to form a lotion. Dab this lotion all over the face and let it dry. Repeat this procedure twice or thrice till the complete lotion has been used up. Helps to remove spots and blemishes if used regularly.

FULLER'S EARTH AND CAMPHOR: Take one tablespoon of fuller's earth and add to it half teaspoon camphor powder and one tablespoon lime juice. Blend well to form a smooth paste. Apply all over the face, rubbing it in gently. Leave it to dry. Rinse and wash off

CARROT PACK: Take 2-3 carrots and grate them after peeling. Boil the grated carrots in very little water till the water dries up. Cool and mash. Apply this pack all over the face. Leave it on for 10-15 minutes; gently rub it in before rinsing off.

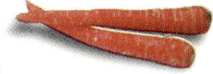

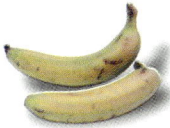

BANANA PACK: An ideal 'food' for the face. It not only nourishes the skin but also 'magically' removes scars, dark patches and blemishes. You will notice the change even after using this once. Take a ripe banana, peel and mash to a pulp. Apply all over the face and leave it on for 10 minutes. Wash off and see your skin come out sparkling clean and nourished. The difference is visible.

39

POTATO PACK: Take a raw potato, peel and grate it. Put the grated potato into a muslin piece and tie it tightly to form a pad. Rub this pad all over the face in firm, circular motions for about 5 minutes and then wash your face. Alternatively you could directly rub potato slices all over your face. Helps to clear blemishes and scars.

COCONUT OIL AND CAMPHOR: In case of minor burns that leave scars, this is a good recipe. Take 2 tablespoons of coconut oil and add to it one teaspoon of camphor powder. Rub thoroughly into the burn mark or scar at least 10 minutes before your bath. Use regularly for quick results. There will be a marked lightening of the scar after a few days.

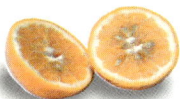

DRIED ORANGE PEELS: Take a few dried orange peels and powder them. Add 2 tablespoons of curd to make a thick paste. Apply all over the face, leaving aside the eye area. Let it dry, then wash thoroughly with cold water. Helps remove blemishes and scars.

FRECKLES

Unevenly distributed melanin (pigmentation) occurs due to exposure to the sun. People who have a fine textured skin and a fair complexion usually get freckles. You should not get unduly upset. Never try and cover up the freckles with makeup, that will only make matters worse. You can certainly try and lighten them.

LEMON, ORANGE OR LIME JUICE: The juice of any one of these can be mixed with a little beaten yoghurt. This paste should be regularly applied on the face and left to dry. Rinse off with cold water. This will help to lighten the freckles.

RADISH: Radish contains a bleaching agent. So take one radish, grate it and add to it the juice of one lime. Blend well and apply all over the face. Leave to dry and then wash off. It not only lightens the freckles but also removes blackheads. Rub vigorously before washing to remove the blackheads.

MINT AND BANANA: Take a few mint leaves and grind them to a paste. Add to this one mashed banana and blend in a blender.

40

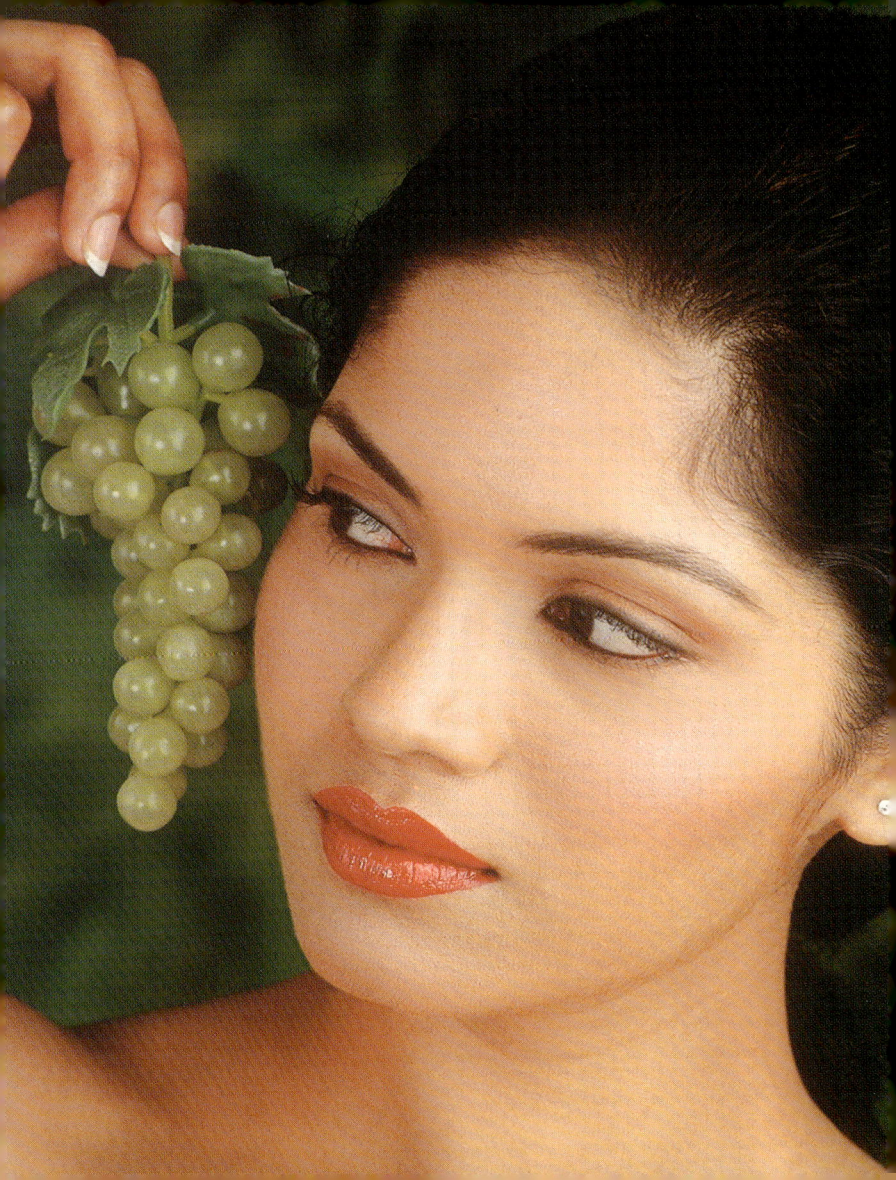

Apply this paste all over the face — be careful to avoid the eyes. Regular use will lighten the freckles and remove blemishes too.

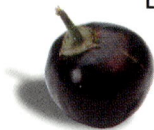

EGGPLANT: Take an eggplant and slice it. Apply fresh eggplant slices all over the freckles, keep rubbing them in a circular motion and leave them on for a few minutes. Use this treatment daily and the results will show after a week.

CRANBERRY AND STRAWBERRY: Rub freshly crushed cranberries or strawberries on your face. Leave the juices and the mashed fruit on your face to dry. Then rinse with cold water. Regular use will lighten the freckles.

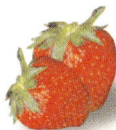

LEMON JUICE AND BORIC ACID: Dissolve one teaspoon boric acid in a cupful of hot water, and add to it the juice of one lemon. Add 2 tablespoons of rose water and half tablespoon of glycerine. Mix well and store this solution in a jar. Dab this lotion on the freckles with a cotton wool pad. Leave it on and later, rinse with water. Regular use will lighten the freckles. If the same solution is rubbed on the neck and shoulders, it makes them fairer, as they usually appear darker than the face.

SUNBURN AND TAN

Having a clear, glowing suntanned skin is the desire of most women. True, the rays of the sun are an essential revitaliser, the sun rays are good for the body as they help in the formation of vitamin D; however, over-exposure to the rays of the sun can also lead to many problems. It can cause sunburn, and other serious problems if the exposure is long and sustained. It can cause redness, sores and even blistering. Thus, some people with delicate skin types need to use a good and effective suntan oil. In cases of over-exposure, tanning and sunburn, here are a few excellent remedies.

CUCUMBER AND MILK: Take a cucumber, skin it and chop it finely and put it in a blender. Make a puree and add one tablespoon of chilled milk. Mix well and apply all over the face, neck, arms and areas scorched or burnt by the sun. Leave on for 15 minutes, and then rinse with cold water. Repeat this treatment twice or thrice during the course of the day. Its soothes the skin and helps in alleviating sunburn.

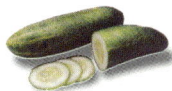

VINEGAR AND WATER: Take 2 tablespoons vinegar and add 2 tablespoons of water. This solution is an ideal cure for suntan. Dab on gently with cotton wool over sore areas. Leave it on for 10 minutes and wash off.

ONION: Take 2 onions, skin and chop them fine. Put then in a mixer and grind to a paste. Tie this in a muslin cloth and squeeze out the juice. Add to the juice a pinch of salt and a tablespoon of milk. Take cotton wool pads and dab over the sunburned or tanned areas. Leave to dry.

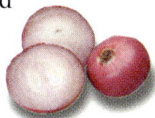

43

Dab the juice again and repeat till the complete solution is used up. Let it dry on your skin. Rinse with cold water. It's best that you make it a routine after coming in from the hot sun.

CUCUMBER AND TOMATO WRAP: Take 2 tomatoes, puree them. Take a cucumber, peel and puree them too. Mix the purees and add to it the juice of one lemon. Mix well. Apply this paste all over the suntanned and sunburnt skin. Let it dry. Dab the puree again. Repeat 3 times and let it dry thoroughly, then rinse off. Use this treatment for a week and see the difference. It not only helps to soothe the burnt area, it adds a glow to the skin too.

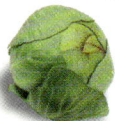

CABBAGE: Take a handful of cabbage leaves, boil them and drain out the water. Mash the leaves and apply the pulp all over the tanned and sunburnt areas. Leave on for 15 minutes. Wash off with cold water. Repeat this treatment at least for a week. This acts like a protective and soothing balm. Use whenever you have been exposed to the hot sun.

GREEN GOURD: Cut green gourd into thin round slices. Rub quickly all over the affected areas. Repeat 3-4 times. Leave it on and wash off at bedtime. Soothes burnt skin.

TUMERIC POWDER AND MILK: Take 3 tablespoons of milk and add to it one tablespoon of turmeric powder. Apply all over the face or affected areas.

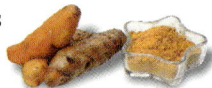

Leave it to dry. Rub in circular motions and then rinse off. It not only helps to remove tan it also helps remove fine facial hair too.

ALOE VERA: The most natural and soothing cure for sunburn and tan. Just pluck a few leaves of the plant, mash or puree them. Add the juice of one lemon. Apply this jelly like solution all over the affected areas. It cleanses, clears and nourishes the skin.

ICE: Use ice cubes all over the sunburned skin when you come from the hot sun.

HONEY AND LIME: Take 2 tablespoons of honey and add to it the juice of one lime. Mix well apply over the sunburned or tanned skin areas. Helps to lighten and soothe the skin.

TOMATO AND OATMEAL: Puree 2 tomatoes. Add 2 tablespoons of curd and one tablespoon of oatmeal or wheat porridge. Mix to a smooth paste. Apply all over suntanned or sunburnt skin. Leave it on for 20 minutes and wash off with cold water. Helps in exfoliation too.

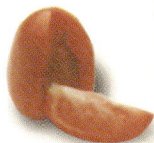

LEMON AND SUGAR: Take the juice of one lemon and add to it a few grains of sugar. Rub this lotion all over the sunburned or tanned areas. Keep rubbing in circular motions. Let it dry and then wash off. This not only helps to remove tan but exfoliates the skin very gently too.

Wrinkles

An ageing skin requires a lot of care, a proper diet and a good exercise regimen to retain youthfulness. Women all over the world fear the onset of wrinkles. They can go to extreme lengths to try and hide, camouflage and delay the process.

Thankfully, there are several natural cures. A proper diet of vegetables, fruits and herbs along with skin-nourishing cures not only delay wrinkles but also improve the texture of your skin. The use of such natural products does not lead to any side effects.

A word of caution too. Your attitude also determines how and when you get wrinkles. Frowning, knitting of the eyebrows, getting easily agitated causes the facial muscles to get tense and knotted up. This too contributes to early wrinkling. Cheer up, there are several simple cures that help. Smiling helps you relax your muscles too.

An ageing skin should take in plenty of fresh fruits and raw salads and yoghurt. The intake of liquids and water should increase manifold. We generally do not drink enough water.

YOGHURT AND CHICKPEA POWDER: Take half cup yoghurt and add 2 tablespoons of chickpea powder. Stir to a smooth paste. Apply a thick coat all over the face and neck. Let it stand for 10 minutes. Wash off. Repeat this every alternate day. This helps to tighten and nourish the skin.

APPLE: If you can use green apples there's nothing better. However any types of apples will also work wonders. Deseed and

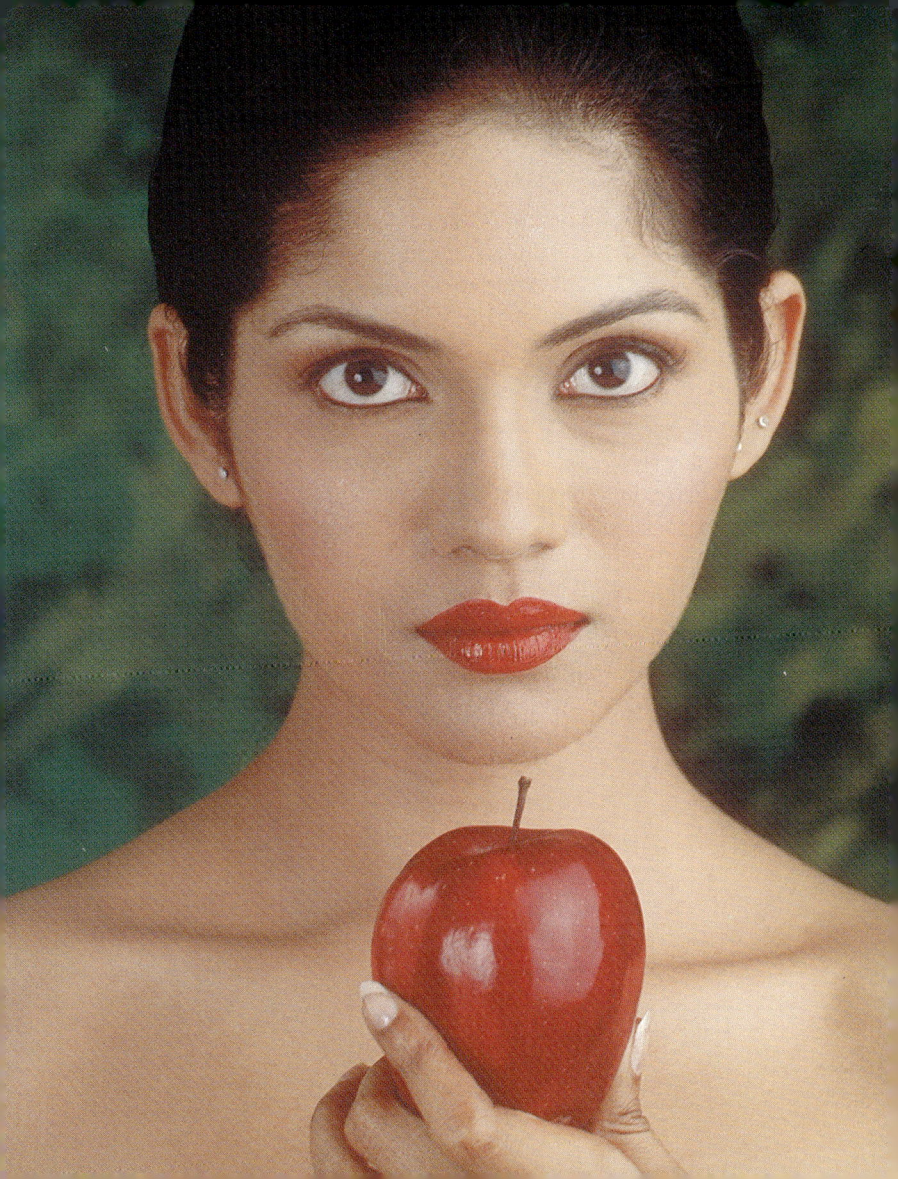

then puree an apple along with its skin. Add one tablespoon of milk and blend well. Apply this apple paste all over the face and neck. Keep taking more of the paste and massage well into the wrinkles. When it begins to dry up, rinse it off.

GLYCERINE AND EGG: This is an effective and an ideal anti wrinkle lotion. Especially good for wrinkles on the hands and the neck. Take the white of an egg in a bowl and add to it 2 tablespoons of glycerine and 2 tablespoons of rose water. Stir well and then apply this lotion on the wrinkled skin as well as on the neck. Sit still and leave it on for 10-12 minutes. Rinse and wash off with cold water. An ideal application.

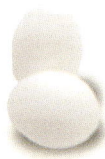

HONEY: Honey works like magic too. A mature skin that has been exposed to the sun and the wind can greatly benefit with this cure. Take 2 tablespoons of honey and to it, add the juice of an orange. Mix well and spread this all over your face and neck. Leave it on for 20 minutes. Gently wipe off with cotton wool dipped in milk. Use this treatment once a day, preferably at bedtime.

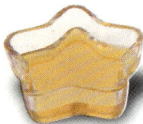

CABBAGE: Take enough cabbage leaves to give you half cup of cabbage juice extract. Add half teaspoon of wet yeast and one tablespoon of honey. Stir to a smooth paste and apply to the face and the neck. Sit still and relax, without making any facial movements. Let the paste dry up. When dry, wash off with lukewarm water.

48

CARROT: Grate 2 carrots and add enough milk to make a thick, non-dripping paste. Spread it evenly all over the face, forehead and the neck. Leave it on for 20 minutes then wash off. This mask rejuvenates the skin.

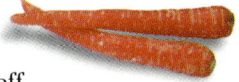

Another very effective mask can be made with grated carrots and egg yolk. Add beaten egg yolk to the grated carrots and add one teaspoon of almond or olive oil. Mix well in a blender to form a smooth paste. Apply all over the forehead, face and neck. Leave it on for 15 minutes. Use cotton wool dipped in warm milk to wipe it off, follow with a rinse.

RICE FLOUR: Take a cup of rice powder and to this add enough milk and rosewater to make a thick paste. Apply evenly all over the forehead, face and the neck area. Leave it on for at least 20 minutes. Try and relax and not move any facial muscles when this paste is applied on the face. After 20-30 minutes when it cakes up, splash cold water on your face, rinse and wash off. The skin appears very taut and the wrinkles seem to have "straightened" out or disappeared altogether. Use this treatment regularly, twice or thrice a week for best results.

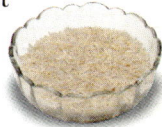

APRICOT: Wrinkles due to tiredness or tension are quickly removed with this wonderful treatment. Take 2 apricots, after de-seeding them, finely chop and puree along with their skin. Add 2

tablespoons of honey and the juice of one lime along with a little cold milk. Blend all these to form a smooth paste. Apply on the forehead, face and the neck. Leave it on for at least 30 minutes. Now take some lukewarm water in a basin and add to it the juice of one lemon. Wash your face with this water. Your face glows and radiates freshness. The worry and furrow lines are minimized. The apricot nourishes while the lime juice tightens the skin.

EGG AND LIME: Take an egg white and beat it well to form peaks. Now add to it the juice of one lime and blend well. Apply all over the forehead, face and neck. Leave it on for 10 minutes. Wash off with lukewarm water. Tightens the skin instantly.

50

GREEN GRAPES: Green seedless grapes are also an excellent cure for wrinkles. Roughly crush a few green seedless grapes and apply them on the forehead, face and neck. Rub the grapes in circular motions on all these areas. Leave them on for 20 minutes. Rinse off with water. Regular use controls wrinkles.

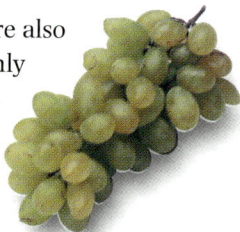

POTATO: A potato mask effectively improves the skin texture, lightens wrinkles, makes them fainter, and tightens your skin. Take 2 potatoes, peel and grate them. Apply the grated potatoes

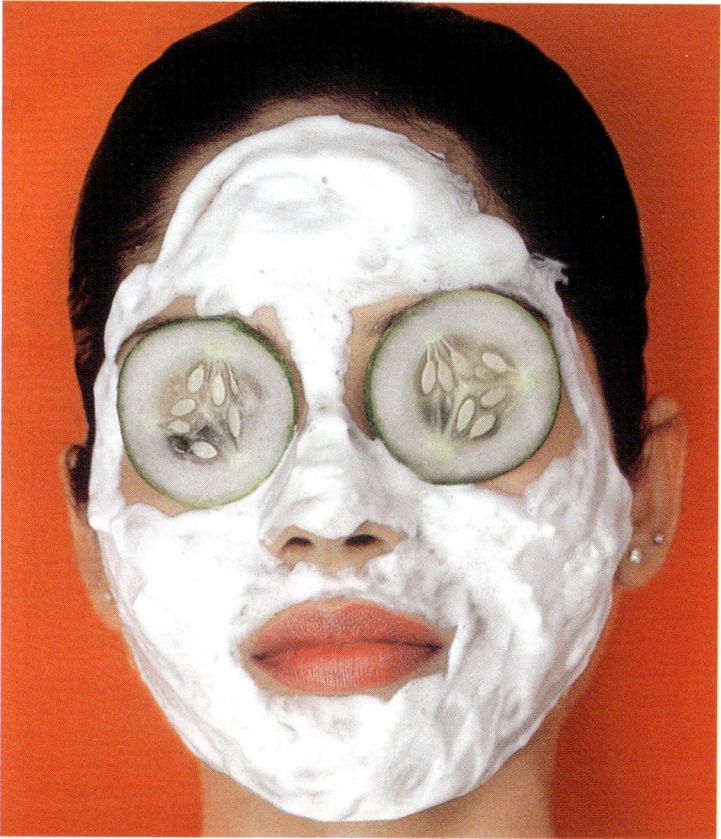

all over forehead, face and neck. Leave it on for a few minutes. The feeling of "pinching" and tightening of the skin will be acute. Rinse off with cold water. Cleans and tightens the skin.

Helpful Tips

You can improve your looks at any age. Equipped with useful tips, a careful diet and regular exercise, you can make your face glow with health, beauty, and vitality; without having to resort to camouflage techniques. Face care varies with skin type. Here are some useful tips.

- Dry skin needs hydrating and moisturizing treatment.
- Oily skin needs cleansing and freshening.
- Patchy skin needs smoothening and lightening treatment.
- Change in season requires a change in the skin care routine.
- To keep the skin glowing, drink at least 12-15 glasses of water per day.
- Your diet should be rich in raw vegetables and fresh fruits. These hydrate your skin.
- Protect yourself from the harshness of the sun. This is the main cause of skin discolouration, pigmentation and wrinkles.
- Exercise regularly; even a good walking routine will suffice.
- Exercise facial muscles regularly. Rotate your neck slowly, side to side, and loosen the facial muscles.
- Laugh loudly, it helps to exercise the facial muscles.
- Wash your face several times a day.

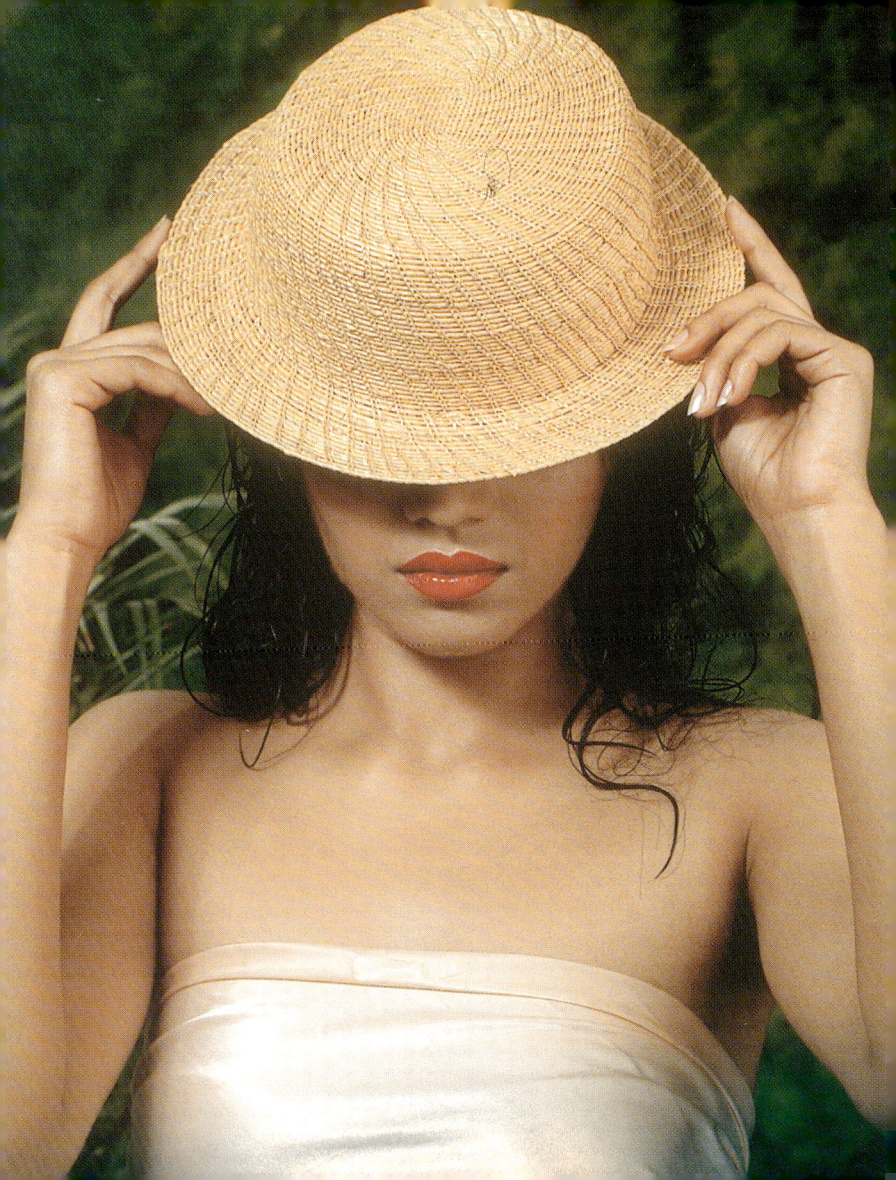

- Steam your face once a week to clean up clogged pores. After steaming, rub your face, forehead and neck vigorously to exfoliate the skin.
- Take Vitamin E for shadows and scars. But consult a doctor first.
- Once a fortnight go in for an elaborate cleansing and moisturizing treatment by using any of the fruits and vegetables mentioned earlier. The type and the nature of the treatment depends upon your skin type.
- "Feed" your skin. It requires nourishment too.
- Whenever you apply a lotion or cream or moisturizer, use gentle swift, featherlike upward strokes. Do not use downward strokes or pull your facial muscles downward, else they will start sagging.
- Whenever you dry your face, always pat it dry. DO NOT RUB, SCRUB OR PULL YOUR SKIN.
- Avoid rapid or excessive weight loss.
- Ensure a good night's sleep. It rests and nourishes your skin.
- A diet rich in Vitamin A prevents a patchy, dry or rough skin. It is also good for people who have acne and pimples.
- Vitamin B prevents spots on the face.
- Strawberries are an instant cure for dry skin. Take a few strawberries, puree them. Add to this half cup milk and a tablespoon of glycerine. Shake well, pour in a jar and store in the refrigerator. Use this whenever the skin appears to be dry and

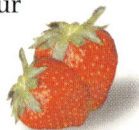

taut. Apply on face, leave on for 10 minutes. Rinse. The skin is as soft like that of a baby.

❀ Your face is the most expressive, noticeable and also the most delicate part of the body. Normal facial expressions like frowning, raising of the eyebrows, wrinkling of the forehead, all this eventually lead to wrinkles. So make a facial massage as a regular routine to combat wrinkling.

❀ Use a moisturizer after exfoliation. It helps to reseal the skin and protects it from over drying.

❀ Prolonged use of alcohol based perfumes and deodorants can cause brown patches and dryness.

❀ Avoid going out in the direct sun when using a perfume. Spray onto clothes instead of on the skin.

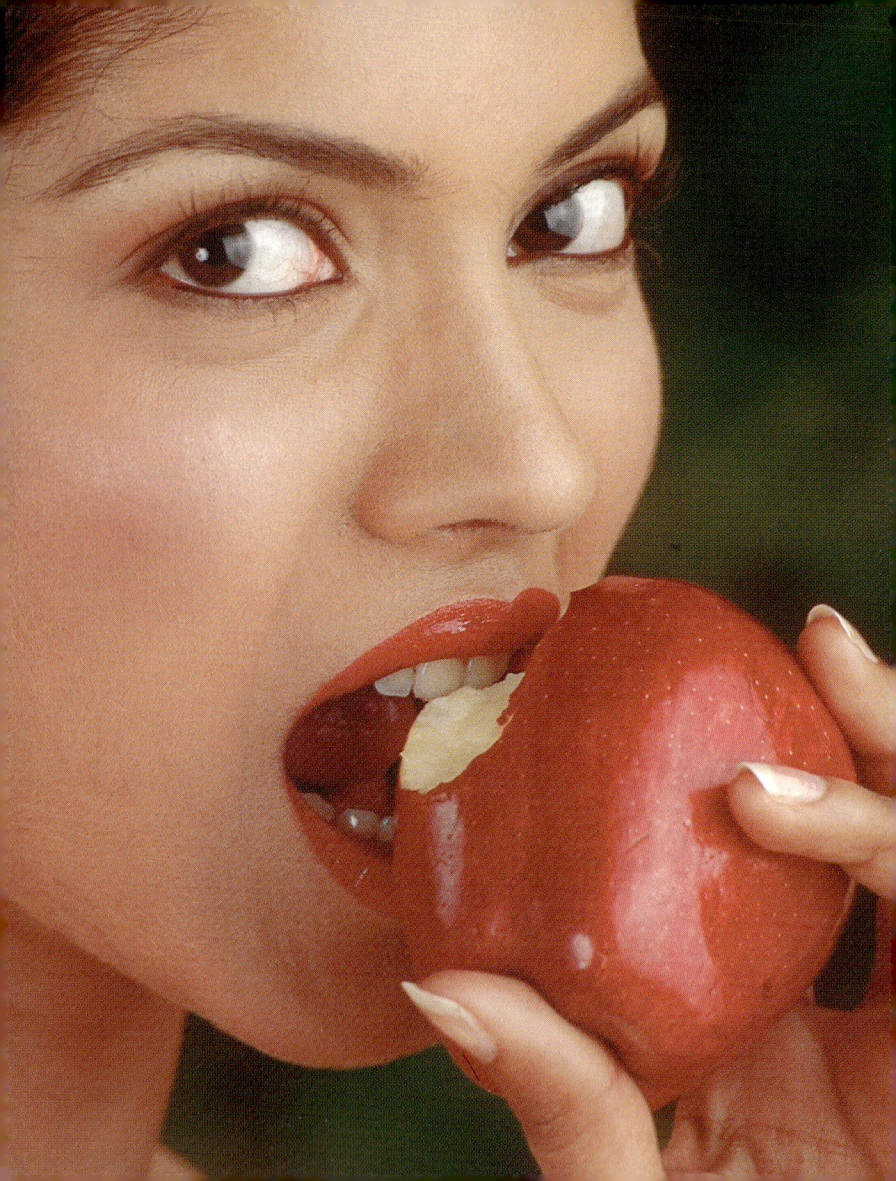

Eat and Grow Beautiful

Looking beautiful and retaining one's beauty should not make you an obsessive slave to beauty cures. While the right use of make-up and beauty care products can undoubtedly enhance your beauty, you can be truly beautiful only if you are healthy. So, eat the right food and grow beautiful. Once you gain knowledge about the right kinds of foods for good health, you can start eating a well-regulated diet, and the results will only be too evident. Your face will glow with health and vitality, your hair will bounce and shine, and your body will be taut and trim. It makes a lot of sense to care not only about the food you eat, but also in the manner in which you do so. A few tips on practical knowledge about food and eating habits would certainly go a long way into developing a healthy regime, which will stand you in good stead.

Undoubtedly, beauty is also a state of the mind. In order to look good, you ought to "feel good" too. True beauty comes from within; from a feeling of well-being. It is not the way you dress, or do your make-up, nor your sense of style or get up, but it is the person within you that looks radiant and beautiful.

Good looks have a lot more to do with food than is commonly realized. The key to vitality, health and beauty is in eating right.

Women in general, and working women in particular, ignore their basic food requirements, leading to malnourishment and other deficiencies. Today, in any urban environment, as much as 75% of young working women are anaemic. This also results in period cramps, heavy bleeding, abdominal bloating and irritability. All this takes a heavy toll on your body and in the way you look. Coupled with this is the fact that many urban women are prone to emotional dieting fads, which messes up the delicate balance within the body, and deprive themselves of essentials like iron, calcium, proteins and minerals. Eventually, this affects the hair, skin, and teeth, and gives the appearance of premature ageing. Bulimia and Anorexia are also growing as women look to magazines and glossy ads and try to be like the thin emasculated models that promote the business of beauty.

Excess of carbohydrates for instance, can take a toll on the hair, skin and the eyes. On the flip side, the addition of vitamins and other nutrients to food can make a difference in the quality of your skin, your hair, and remove headaches and irritability and other day-to-day ailments. Did you know that sluggishness and lack of energy could be overcome with a changed and improved diet plan?

All this does not imply that you need to be fastidious or obsessive about your food. It only means that you need to have basic nutritional awareness about your food. You can thus select the right kinds of foods best suited to the needs of your body. Its your daily food intake that is important. So, do spare a thought for food. Make sure that you get enough nutrients and have a balanced diet. This is the key to good health and beauty. Modern day eating habits, convenient cooking and fast food culture robs us of essentials like vitamin B complex, as found in milk, liver, fish and wheat germ. We tend to cultivate wrong eating habits. Let me just tell you very briefly about some nutrients that are absolutely essential for a sound and healthy body.

Skin: Your skin needs Vitamin B2. This is present in fresh vegetables, milk, whole wheat bread. It also needs Vitamin C to

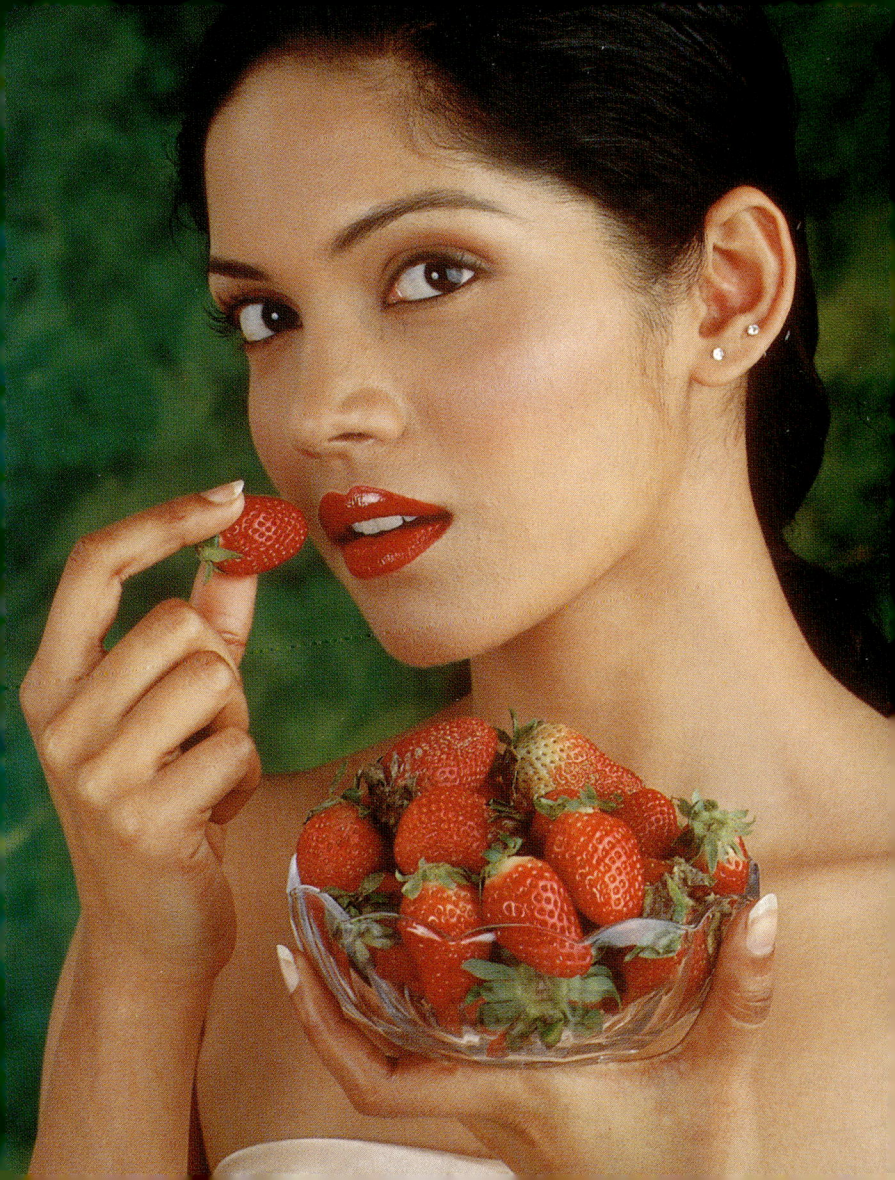

vitalize and purify the bloodstream. The easy way out? Eat at least one orange a day. Simple!

Teeth and Bones: These need calcium and Vitamin D. So take plenty of milk and fish. Avoid too much of starch and sugar. This builds healthy and strong teeth and bones.

Hair: Hair is made from a protein-based substance called keratin. Thus, a healthy mane of hair needs plenty of protein and vitamin B. A high protein diet should include fish, cheese and eggs.

Nails: To avoid chipping, cracking and discolouring of nails, ensure that you have a diet rich in proteins and minerals and iodine.

Eyes: The most essential requirement for healthy eyes is Vitamin A. Carrots and cabbage and other leafy vegetables are a good source, as are butter, eggs and fish.

Over the years, our eating habits have deteriorated. Coupled with the fact that pesticides are being used in grains, fruits and vegetables, eventually they rob you of essential "natural" nutrients. Today's working women seek a quick and easy way out. Thus, many people go in for processed foods, which may be the primary cause of poor nutrition. There is really no substitute for nature. We have seen it time and again. Natural produce, fruits, vegetables and food grains are best when grown in its natural process without any artificial ingredients. An increasingly large number of people are depriving themselves of essential nutrients. True, the modern, stressful lifestyle may be a cause, but lack of interest and ignorance about the basic nutritional values is definitely the other cause.

In today's lifestyle, busy people with little time for shopping for food and even lesser time for cooking it, do not realise the harmful effects of only relying on processed foods. Besides, the marketing hype and fashion cults often change, dictate and shape people's food habits. Be wary of such sensationalism. Do not become a prey to these superficial swings in food habits, for they are based on economics and your health is never the consideration. A bit of intuitive know how and a lot of commonsense can steer you to a healthy way of eating for a more beautiful you.

One of the most glaring bad food habits that exist today is subsistence on hastily prepared foods or convenience foods as they are called. These are semi-processed add-some-water-type of preparations. Thus, essential minerals are robbed from your food. Today's staple diet consists of foods that are used as snacks. Lack of time, or rather the lack of priority in one's life are the reasons why one so often picks up bad eating habits. If you plan ahead, and educate yourself about the nutritive values of common day-to-day food products, you can eat well and grow beautiful. Let your body "talk" about the food it needs.

There is also a need to dispel some myths about food, nutrients and diet. Some believe that the key to health and beauty is by increasing the daily dose of vitamins. So popping pills becomes a common everyday occurrence. You may not even need to take pills unless you are short on any particular vitamin that you may need to supplement. Mindless pill popping is harmful. Excess is worse than deficiency.

Your Kitchen
A Treasure Trove

Nature has been very generous with its bounty of fruits, flowers, vegetables and herbs. It gives us all that we need to look beautiful, remain healthy and stay youthful.

Plants have provided man with his total needs. Foods that sustain us and help us to remain healthy. Vitamins and minerals that meet the total needs of the body. Fruits, vegetables and herbs that give a special sparkle to the eyes; luster to the hair and colour to the cheeks.

The early Egyptians were the first to take an interest in using plants for making perfumes and cosmetics. They perhaps learnt the art from the Mesolithic travellers who roamed the Nile valley in 5,000 to 10,000 BC.

The Egyptians had a cure and a preparation for every part of the body. Ancient Egyptian women improved and enhanced their appearances with a variety of cosmetics made from the Earth's bounty.

A judicious use of nature's gifts helps you to enhance your assets and improve upon your drawbacks. It certainly makes you aware that beauty and health are intertwined. Good nutrition and use of natural beauty aids can radiate that aura of beauty that was dormant within you. With the use of these fruits, vegetables, flowers and herbs, you can improve the quality of your hair, texture of your skin and in fact rejuvenate yourself completely.

Health and confidence will reflect not only on your face but also in your complete personality. So, go ahead and make yourself beautiful, not by putting layers of make-up but by enhancing the quality of your skin; hair, and complexion. And by, being content and happy with the way you look naturally. Be beautiful and happy from within.

We owe it to ourselves to spend a little time and effort to grow beautiful. Equipped with these helpful hints from skincare; hair care, face care to nutritional guidelines, you can discover ways to improve your looks and remain youthful and beautiful.

Before you decide on a course of self-improvement, you first need to do a thorough body-check. Recognize your weak beauty points and set about the task of improving upon them and enhancing them. Every product cannot give you a miraculous cure. Using products to improve and enhance yourself has to be a determined and deliberate effort, and it has to fit into a normal routine of your lifestyle. Decide what is best for you; what enhancers you really need and then go about using them regularly to show results and maintain them.

When you are young, you have enough time and spare cash to look after yourself. But as you take on responsibilities of home, hearth and children, beauty care need not take a back seat for want of time or money, if you use the products so easily available in your own kitchen.

Today, beauty houses the world over are being compelled to go back to nature; to use more natural products in their preparations. The modern woman is going back to nature, both in her eating habits and for her body care. Homemade natural beauty aids can prove to be effective if used correctly and consistently.

As you would have realized after going through the beauty care suggestions; fruits, flowers, herbs and vegetables provide cures for improving the quality of the skin, giving a glow to a tired face, imparting health, colour and body to your hair, thus imparting a sense of well-being to the complete body. True, these beauty cures do not have a shelf life, as they contain no preservatives or chemicals. However, you just need to analyse what you need to use everyday, or every week. Once you establish a routine, the task of making and using them is worth the effort of making them fresh. So, spare a little time for yourself.

Let us now take a look at what your beauty treasure trove in the kitchen has to offer. Indeed your kitchen is like an eco-friendly cosmetic laboratory. It provides you with beauty aids for almost every problem and helps you to overcome flaws, if any, and to enhance your beauty. These cures usually have no side effects and instead beautify you from within and not merely superficially.

Let us now recapitulate some of the most easily available beauty cure aids available right here in your kitchen:

ALMOND: The juice of Almonds, crushed and powdered almonds are extensively used to make face packs, skin nourishers and night creams that nourish and 'feed' your skin. They are extremely useful on aged or wrinkled skins. Usually mixed with rose water and glycerin to make skin nourishers. When added to milk, makes an excellent mask that nourishes and softens your skin.

APPLE: Apple juice if mixed with Vinegar makes an excellent hair rinse. Grated apple paste mixed with honey or milk makes an excellent facemask, very useful for complexion cures.

APRICOT: Fresh apricots blended with honey or milk; or fresh apricot paste by itself makes excellent face-masks, which is a very effective nourisher for dry skin, chapped arms, and it helps in rejuvenating dead skin.

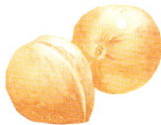

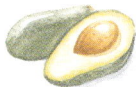

AVOCADO: This is a universal favourite. The pulp of this fruit is a skin nourisher and provides an excellent 'food' for the skin. If added to honey or curds, it makes an excellent moisturizer.

BANANA: Pulp if mixed with milk, honey or curds makes a good face-mask that rids you of blemishes. An excellent skin softener. Pulp when mixed with curd and beaten to a thick paste is excellent for your hair, promotes healthy, glossy hair and gives them a unique shine.

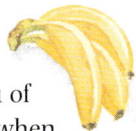

CARROT: The ideal 'wrinkle fighter'. Raw carrots grated and added to almond oil and honey and applied as a thick mask, fights wrinkles.

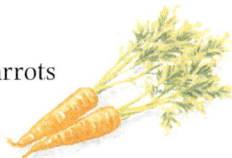

CHICKPEA POWDER: Used as a base for different types of face-masks and as a skin softener and exfoliate. It helps to remove dead skin; hair on the arms and blemishes as well as acne.

COCONUT OIL: Used in numerous beauty care aids. Excellent hair nourisher.

CUCUMBER: Some of the best skin preparations are made from cucumber. When used with curds, makes good, nourishing complexion masks. When used by itself, its juices remove dark circles and blemishes. An excellent skin tauter; it also closes pores, fights skin tan and helps in rejuvenating the skin.

GARLIC: Good for its medicinal properties. If taken raw, it purifies the blood, thus giving a clearer complexion. It also heals cuts and wounds, and clears blemishes if its juice is applied.

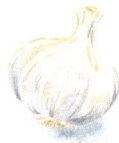

GRAPEFRUIT: When the fruit is blended with yogurt it makes a good skin tonic. A skin tautner that also cures blemishes and shadows.

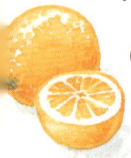

HONEY: A pre-requisite for so many skin nourishers; face-masks and skin tonics. If taken daily with lime and warm water, it purifies blood and clears the skin of blemishes.

HENNA: Its leaves are dried and powdered. Used not only to decorate and beautify the palms, it is universally used as a hair conditioner, colorant and nourisher.

LAVENDER: Its flowers are used to make soaps and hair creams. the oils in these flowers promote hair growth. You can make excellent toilet waters from it to soothe tired nerves. Its essential oils are excellent coolants for headaches and migraines.

LEMON: One of the most commonly used ingredients. A perfect all-rounder used for removing skin tans; as a facemask; as an astringent, as a skin toner and lightener. It tautens the skin and removes wrinkles. Useful to fight dandruff and an excellent tonic if imbibed with honey.

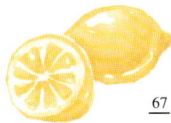

67

LILAC: Its flowers not only yield a wonderful perfume, they make excellent astringents, bath waters, and soothe sunburnt skin.

MARIGOLD: Its flowers are used to make face creams and skin ointments. It is soothing to the eyes too.

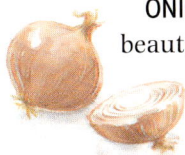

ONION: Onion juice can again be used in various beauty cure treatments. Its juice cures pimples, burn scars and is excellent for dandruff problems. It also helps to restore natural hair colour.

OATS: An excellent base for making face packs, exfoliates and is a remarkable skin tightener.

OLIVE: Used to prepare skin creams to nourish the skin. Revives jaded skin and good for dull, lifeless hair.

PAPAYA: Again, an excellent and commonly used base for face packs and an excellent hair conditioner. It adds bounce and shine to the hair. The papaya is easily available and its regular use does wonders for your skin and hair.

PEACH: An all time favourite with beauticians all over the world. Makes nourishing facemasks and packs. Fights dry skin and curbs wrinkles. Exfoliates and nourishes.

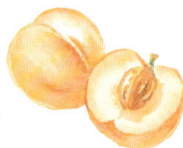

POTATO: A remarkable skin tautner and helps lighten tan. Heals burns, cuts and lightens your complexion. Helps to get rid of burn marks, removes pimples and freckles.

ROSE: Its petals are used to make a number of beauty preparations and astringents. It softens the skin, fights dry chapped skin and soothes jaded skin.

SAFFRON: Skin enhancer and softener. Excellent for the complexion.

68

SAGE: Used as a hair colorant. If used with olive oil it also nourishes dry, lifeless hair.

SANDALWOOD: Commonly associated with making perfumes. Its powder when mixed with honey or milk enhances the skin miraculously. It fights tanning; softens the skin and is an excellent cure for pimples, blackheads and blemishes.

STRAWBERRY: Its fruit is crushed and used with milk or honey to make facemasks. Just strawberry juice by itself is an ideal cure for clearing blemishes.

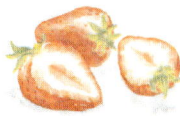

SUNFLOWER: This is also used to cure blemishes.

TUMERIC: Has tremendous curative powers. Cures scars and burn marks. It smoothens the skin and is a base for many other tonics.

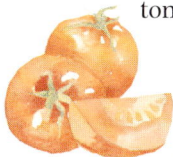

TOMATO: Another favourite 'skin toner'. Makes good facemasks. A good cleanser and useful for clearing the skin of marks and blemishes.

WALNUT: Both the fruit and its shell are used to darken the hair. Oils extracted from these are used as hair darkeners and mixed with shampoo to give a sheen and gloss and volume to the hair.

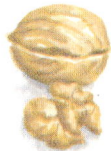

WATERCRESS: Used to clear the skin. It smoothens the skin. A paste made from this when applied on burn marks clears them quickly. A good skin hydrator.

WATERMELON: An ideal skin hydrator. It makes the skin taut, refreshed and rehydrated. It also helps to clear shadows under the eyes. There is no better moisturizer than watermelon.

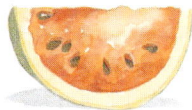

WHEAT: Its husk, or porridge are good exfoliates. Also used as a base in a number of skin mask preparations.

LETTUCE: Makes an excellent astringent. Fights acne and blemishes.

YOGURT: Used in numerous skin preparations to make skincare masks packs, and by itself as a skin smoothener. Fights acne. Yogurt is also used in a number of hair care preparations. It nourishes the hair, helping in healthy hair growth.

The magical beauty treasure chest in your own kitchen can help you create your own beauty kit. You can remain beautiful and healthy by using these natural beauty aids. Ultimately, we do fall back on nature to help us become truly beautiful. So give yourself a natural makeover from your own kitchen beauty box, which is indeed a treasure trove of beauty aids.